^{to}BURN_{or not}
^{to}BURN

FAT

is the question

to BURN or not to BURN

FAT

is the question

Len Lopez, DC, CCN

BROWN BOOKS PUBLISHING GROUP
DALLAS, TEXAS

To Burn or Not to Burn, FAT is the Question
Copyright © 2003 Dr. Len Lopez
Printed in the United States of America
ISBN 0-9710797-1-4

Photographer: Mandy Johnson
Designer: Alyson Alexander
Illustrator: Pete Grubb

Brown Books Publishing Group
16200 Dallas Parkway, Suite 170
Dallas, Texas 75248
972-381-0009
www.brownbooks.com

www.DrLenLopez.com

The information and advice contained in this book are based upon the author's personal and professional experiences and are not intended to replace proper medical advice. Before beginning any health program, you should consult with your health care provider. The author is not responsible for any adverse effects resulting from the use of any principles discussed in this book.

Dedication

I dedicate this book to the memory of my father, Frank R. Lopez Jr., one of the greatest men I have ever known.

From your humble beginnings, Dad, I will always remember the smile on your face and the joy you took in telling a story. You were strict with three boys, but you raised us with love. You taught my brothers and me so much about life—the importance of family and sacrifice—not by words but by action.

It's been said the greatest gift you can give your kids is to love their mother. Dad, thank you for the forty-seven years of marriage to our mom. We don't have you to lead this family any longer, but I know our Lord has plans that we don't understand. I know you are looking down at us right now with a big, proud smile. Thank you for all your sacrifice and devotion to our family; we are going to miss you, so very, very much.

Your Middle Son,

Len

Table of Contents

Introduction

If you are one of the millions of people who constantly struggle with your weight and are always on some type of diet or exercise program to help fight the battle of the bulge, this book will be very helpful to you.

Many people spend half their lives dieting, yet they still can't lose any weight. Some wonder why they spend so much time exercising with little or no results to show. Others claim they do a good job of dieting and exercising, but are still unable to reach their desired weight loss goals. With so much dieting and exercise, we should be seeing more positive results. Unfortunately, here in America, problems with weight gain and obesity are a growing concern and never-ending problem for many.

Most people think diet and exercise are all that's involved when it comes to losing weight and keeping it off. There are many people who diet properly and routinely exercise but are still not seeing the results they want when they look in the mirror. Keep in mind that if you are dieting properly and routinely exercise but still not losing weight or shaping up, then diet and exercise may not be the only pieces of this puzzle. There could be another factor we haven't looked at before. Stress!

Stress may be part of the problem that's holding back your results. Is there heavy stress in your life? Do you always feel fatigued and run down? Are you constantly on the go? Do you suffer from headaches, indigestion, bloating, constipation, allergies, PMS, menopause, arthritis, diabetes, and/or low blood sugar? Do you not get enough sleep each night? If you're answering yes to this short list of questions there is a good chance that stress is overwhelming your body and triggering hormonal responses that are working against you in your weight loss efforts. It's also a possibility that your diet and exercise programs may be triggering the wrong hormonal responses. You could be activating all the triggers that promote your body to store fat rather than burn fat.

Burning Calories

All we have heard about for the last 25 years has been how many calories we need to burn to lose weight. What we are starting to realize is that it doesn't necessarily matter how many calories we burn each day if we are always burning calories from the wrong source. Let me explain. The human body can burn calories from carbohydrates, proteins or fats. The biggest problem for most people who are unsuccessful with their weight loss efforts is that they are constantly burning calories from carbohydrates and proteins and not from fats. When you can start triggering your body to burn calories from stored body fat, you will be able to finally succeed in your weight loss efforts.

We have been led to believe that losing weight and keeping it off is only a matter of counting the number of calories we eat in our diet and counting the number of calories we burn in our workout routines. There is more to it than that. Just because the machine you just finished exercising with stated you had burned 300 calories doesn't mean you burned 300 calories from stored body fat. You could have burned 300 calories from all the carbohydrates you just consumed in your last meal.

The key is triggering your body to burn fat and not store fat! This is where our hormones come into play. Hormones regulate our bodies. In fact, they trigger various responses. Some hormones trigger our bodies to burn fat, some hormones trigger our bodies to store fat and some hormones trigger our bodies to burn carbohydrates and proteins. Obviously, if you're trying to lose weight it would be smarter to trigger your body to produce more of the hormones that burn fat rather than storing fat.

This is what you will learn as you read this book. You will learn how stress, diet, and exercise trigger your hormones to either burn or store fat. You will learn which hormones work in your favor and which hormones work against all your dieting efforts. The best part about this whole process of triggering various hormones to work with us is that we have a great deal of control as to which hormones are being produced and how we can regulate them to help us lose weight.

As you read, you will learn the type of diet to follow in order to help produce hormones that will burn fat. You will learn the type of workout routine that will help you burn calories from stored body fat. Most importantly, you will learn the overwhelming effect stress has on your body's ability to either burn or store fat.

Getting Healthy

The final point I want to make known as you read this book is that not only do I want to help you get thinner, I want to help you become healthier. There are a lot of unhealthy skinny people out and about. Fortunately, the suggestions outlined in this book will help us not only lose weight by regulating our hormones in response to our diet, exercise routine, and stress level, but we will also move closer to overall better health.

The one important thing I have learned in almost ten years of clinical practice is that almost everyone who has sought my advice on losing weight usually came with a whole laundry list of other health complaints. Oftentimes patients would also complain of fatigue, headaches, PMS, menopause, cravings, heartburn, indigestion, bloating, gas, constipation, irritability, mood swings, low blood sugar, inability to concentrate, insomnia, arthritis, diabetes, allergies, and other symptoms. What I have learned is that you must take into consideration what all those symptoms mean when designing a diet and exercise program for someone.

We are not all the same, but when our bodies are bombarded with all these symptoms (signals), they are letting us know that something inside isn't working properly. We may have to address some of those symptoms at the same time we are working on our weight loss program. We may still be able to lose weight, but I believe the overall goal should be getting healthier while at the same time getting thinner. The amazing thing is that as we get our bodies healthier and back in balance, it is much easier for the body to drop that unwanted weight.

I want to wish you the best of luck as you strive toward a leaner and healthier body, and I hope you can follow the Actions Steps suggested at the end of each chapter.

Chapter One

Good Health and Good Fitness

Imagine for a moment you are lost in the mountains one night with no supplies and you're only dependent upon yourself for survival. As you search for the right direction to return home safely, you come upon an empty cabin to take shelter in. There is a huge fireplace inside, and you realize the importance of getting a fire started to keep warm through the night. As you search the cabin you joyfully find some matches and three stacks of wood in front of the fireplace. One of the stacks consists of small twigs, another stack is made up of small branches and the third stack, which is the largest, consists of large pieces of chopped wood.

Your goal will be to get a fire started, keep it burning all night, and have it burn hot enough to keep you warm. With that in mind, which of the three stacks of wood do you want to burn? If you have any knowledge about starting a fire, you need the twigs and small branches to get the fire started, but it will be the big logs that will generate the most heat and burn for the longest period of time.

The human body functions much like the fireplace and those different stacks of logs; the body burns calories from carbohydrates, proteins, and fats. Think of those stacks of twigs, small branches, and logs as carbohydrates, proteins, and fats, respectively. If you want to generate the most heat and keep the fire burning for a long period of time, it is important to burn those big fat logs. Losing weight and keeping it off is very similar; you need to make sure your body is burning calories from stored body fat. Sure, you can have a roaring fire burning, but is that red hot fire being generated by nothing but

1

twigs and small branches, or is the heat coming off that blazing fire a result of all those big fat logs that you tossed in the fire?

This is the major problem so many people have when it comes to successfully losing weight—they are constantly burning calories not from stored body fat but instead are burning calories from all the carbohydrates and proteins in their bodies. Our metabolism is constantly burning calories throughout the day, but the key question should be: Are you burning calories from carbohydrates, proteins or fats?

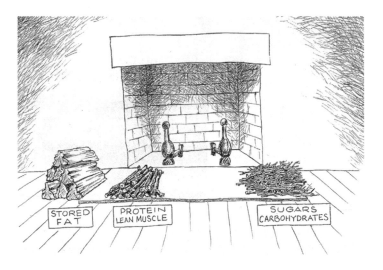

Which calories are you burning?

As we continue with this analogy you will notice there are a few other striking similarities that I think we need to discuss. First, out in the woods, we only stockpile a limited amount of twigs and small branches to burn during the winter. Well, the human body only has a limited supply of carbohydrates and proteins it can burn for calories. Secondly, we need to stockpile as many big fat logs behind the barn to get us through the cold winter. Unfortunately, many of us are stockpiling too many logs (fats) out behind the barn (around our backsides) expecting the winter to last for a long, long time. Now, I say that jokingly because it fits in nicely with my analogy, but the key point I want you to understand is that in order to finally burn those extra pounds we've been struggling with, we need to trigger the appropriate hormones that burn calories from all the stored body fat we've stockpiled over time and quit burning the limited supply of carbohydrates and proteins in our bodies.

We will discuss later how we can trigger our hormones to work with us or against us in our weight loss efforts, but right now I want you to realize there is a limited amount of calories we can burn from carbohydrates and proteins. We can only store a limited amount of carbohydrates in our bodies before they are converted and stored as fat. If we constantly keep triggering our hormones to burn calories from carbohydrates instead of stored body fat you will begin to notice a few symptoms such as food cravings, low blood sugar, irritability, lightheadedness, difficulty concentrating, and the need to eat every few hours in order to keep your blood sugar level.

This is similar to constantly having to keep shoving twigs into the fireplace in order to keep the fire going. Remember, you can have a roaring fire going by only burning twigs and small branches. The problem is that you have to frequently keep throwing twigs into the fire to keep it going, which is a hassle and very inefficient. With that being said, it makes it easier to identify, based on symptoms, who is burning more calories from carbohydrates versus fats.

As we move along to the limited amount of protein or lean muscle tissue we have on our bodies, we must understand that we really don't want to burn calories from proteins. Remember, we have a limited supply of muscle on our bodies and that's the last source of fuel we should be depleting, because the number one bio-marker for aging is percent of lean muscle tissue, which means the more lean muscle tissue we have as we age the better our overall health. Therefore, a classic sign for someone who may be burning calories from proteins instead of fats is the person who never seems to add any shape or tone to his or her body for the amount of hours he or she spends working out. If that sounds like you that can explain why you haven't been able to add that lean muscle tissue to your body.

I would like to kick off our discussion on losing weight and keeping it off by sharing this simple analogy of the fireplace in the woods, because the stumbling block for many people is they simply aren't burning calories from stored body fat. It's not that we're not dieting or exercising, because millions of people are doing all that. Unfortunately, we've gotten so caught up with the notion of burning calories that we have forgotten to ask what the source of all those calories is? When you can continually trigger your body to burn more calories from stored fat than from carbohydrates and proteins, you will finally be able to successfully succeed in your weight loss efforts.

Where To Start

Many people are following some type of diet and/or exercise program without reaching their desired goals of losing weight, keeping it off, and toning up. Why is losing weight and keeping it off such a problem for most people?

Perhaps the reason we can't come up with the right answers to this puzzling question is because we're asking all the wrong questions. There is an old saying that says, "You don't need to have the right answers if you don't ask the right questions." Could it be more than just eating the right amount of calories? Could it be more than just eating the right amount of fats? Could it be more than just exercising that will have an effect on our weight loss efforts? Are those the right questions?

It's obvious the answers we're getting are in many cases not the answers to why we can't seem to successfully lose weight and keep it off. That's why we may need to start asking some different questions, because if we keep asking the same questions we're going to get the same answers. We need to wake up and realize that for the last twenty-five years we have steadily increased the rate of obesity, heart disease, stroke, diabetes, cancer, and the list can go on and on.

We need to start asking some different questions. Maybe it's more than just diet and exercise; maybe there is another piece of the puzzle? Maybe we need to start thinking outside the box and ask some different questions such as:

- Can stress affect whether or not our bodies burn or store fat?
- Can stress be affecting our hormones?
- Do our hormones have an effect on our body weight and metabolism?
- Is the stress in our life affecting the balance of our hormones?
- Is our diet disrupting hormonal balance?
- Can the foods we eat trigger our body to burn or store body fat?
- Does the intensity of our workout or the type of workout have an effect?
- Is it important to just burn calories or do we need to examine where those calories come from?

Most people today only want to concentrate on counting calories, counting fats and keeping track of their exercise programs. In this book we will explore some questions that aren't being asked. This may help many people who have been unsuccessful with their weight loss results, even though they've been dieting and exercising. If you're like most people, you don't want to waste all your time, energy, and efforts dieting and working out without getting the results you want.

As I said earlier, there may be another piece of the puzzle besides diet and exercise that needs to be examined. I believe there are three pieces to the puzzle! Stress and the impact it has on weight loss has been overlooked. Just think about it: if you are unable to lose weight, keep it off, and tone up the body while you are doing all the proper dieting and exercising, what else could it be? We need to examine stress and the effect it has on our hormones and our ability to either store or burn fat.

Regulating Our Hormones Is the Key

It's not just the calories! It's not just the fats! It's not just dependent on what time you eat! Nor is it simply the exercises that you are doing that will determine if your body is going to gain additional weight or not! To achieve long-term and lasting results from any weight loss program we must recognize that our hormones and our ability to regulate them will have a direct impact on our weight loss efforts.

Science has taught us that our hormones regulate everything in our body. In fact, we have learned that some hormones trigger our bodies to burn fats, while other hormones trigger our bodies to store fats. We've learned there are some hormones that trigger our bodies to burn carbohydrates or proteins. Knowing that information should help us in our weight loss efforts, because if you're trying to lose weight, wouldn't it be smarter to make sure your body is triggering the hormones that burn fat and not store fat? The answer to that question is very obvious, but I think the best part of the answer is that we have a great deal of control over those hormones.

We need to understand that the level of stress in our lives will trigger various hormones. The types of foods we eat in our diets and the intensity of our workouts will also trigger various hormones. What I plan to share with you and teach you in the chapters to come are which hormones have a positive effect and which hormones have a negative effect on your weight loss efforts. I also plan to share with you how to regulate those hormones and how to get them in balance with each other.

Many of the hormones we will be speaking about later in the book are produced by our endocrine systems. In simple terms, the thyroid gland produces hormones that regulate our metabolisms, which controls the rate at which our bodies burn calories. However, it is the stress hormones produced by our adrenal glands that may determine if our bodies are going to burn calories from stored body fat, lean muscle tissue, or foods we recently consumed. Are the hormones that our thyroid and adrenal glands produce being properly regulated? Or are they so far out of balance from stress, fad diets, poor nutrition, and lifestyle choices that they are not working for us but rather against us. These could be some of the simple reasons why we don't succeed in our weight loss efforts.

When it comes to diet, the two hormones that need to be discussed are insulin and glucagon. These two hormones are involved in regulating your blood sugar levels, which are very important in controlling your weight. These hormones are triggered in response to what we eat and drink on a daily basis.

Insulin is produced in response to carbohydrates and is considered an anabolic hormone. Anabolic is defined as "to build up" or "to grow." Glucagon, on the other hand, is produced in the absence of carbohydrates and is a catabolic hormone. The definition of catabolic is to break down and tear apart. Is your body producing an equal amount of these two hormones to burn fat and keep your blood sugar level? Does your diet cause you to produce more insulin, which can make you heavier? Do you produce enough glucagon to keep your blood sugar level? Can stress affect how these two hormones operate? Do the food choices you make each day drive your blood sugar levels so far out of balance that it makes it more difficult to succeed in a healthy weight management program?

Lastly, are you getting a good balance of both aerobic and anaerobic training in your schedule? Are you mistakenly doing more of one type of training than the other, which can throw you out of balance? Does one type of training burn more calories from fats than the other? Can the intensity level you train at produce an imbalance of aerobic and anaerobic metabolism? Is your aerobic training triggering aerobic metabolism or is it triggering anaerobic metabolism? Does it matter what type of exercise you do?

These are some of the most essential questions we need to be asking if we are going to look at how stress, diet, and exercise trigger our hormones to burn or store fat. Ask yourself: are your stress level, diet (blood sugar level), and exercise routine working in your favor to promote healthy weight loss? Or, do the stress in your life, the food choices you make, and the type of workout you perform throw your hormones further out of balance and make your body work against you? If you're not triggering your body to burn calories from stored fat, you will always be struggling with your weight.

The great fringe benefit of regulating your hormones as you strive to lose weight and keep it off is that you will become healthier. If you restore balance back to your body and rebalance your hormonal system, you can return your body back to good health. As you restore your body back into a state of good health, you will find that your body doesn't have to hold onto so much extra body fat. A healthy body doesn't need all the excess body fat. All that extra weight places more stress on our bones, muscles, joints, and backs. It makes our hearts work harder and taxes our cardiovascular systems. It affects our breathing, immune systems, respiratory, and cardiovascular system. I can go on and on how this extra weight is taxing your body. Please realize that as you become healthier your ability to keep the weight off will become easier as well.

The Purpose of Diet and Exercise

Most people who diet and exercise simply want to look and feel better each day. Many have stated that if they were happy and content with the way they physically look, they would feel better about themselves. If that's true, most people will start feeling better about themselves once they get their bodies to start looking more physically fit. For some people becoming a little more fit may mean dropping 20–40 pounds. Others may define more fit as keeping their weight the same but firming up their arms and legs. Still others would be happy if they could keep the weight off for more than a few months.

To Burn or Not To Burn, Fat is the Question was written to help people understand that healthy weight loss is not based solely on diet and exercise. Stress can be one of the main contributors to the puzzle! Stress can trigger many hormonal responses that can work against all of our dieting and exercising efforts. My goal is to share with you how constant and excessive daily stress can cause hormonal imbalance and trigger your body to work against you and negate all your dieting and exercising efforts. How we have control over our diet and exercise routines can regulate various hormones to have a positive effect on our bodies.

To achieve healthy weight loss, you need to look not only at diet and exercise but also how stress affects weight loss. In particular, we need to pay attention to the hormonal responses that are triggered from stress, diet, and exercise. Those hormones determine whether or not we are placing logs in our fireplace or just twigs and small branches. This is why counting calories and fat grams may not be the total answer to our weight loss problems. Just because we have a roaring fire constantly burning in our little cabin, don't assume the source of that fire came from all the big logs we have stockpiled. That roaring fire may be the result of twigs and small branches constantly being burned. This is why most people aren't successful at losing weight. They are constantly burning calories from carbohydrates and proteins, not fats. Therefore, be aware if you suffer with low blood sugar, cravings, irritability, moodiness, lightheadedness, inability to concentrate, or the need to eat every few hours, as there is a good chance your body is constantly burning carbohydrates, not fats.

The major underlying theme of this book is to help you become healthier—not just become thinner! There are plenty of skinny, unhealthy people walking around today. My goal is to help you maximize the time, energy, and effort you spend dieting and exercising, while at the same time promote better health.

The three pieces of the puzzle (stress, diet, and exercise), we will explore are all very important. The first topic we will discuss will be the effects stress has on our hormonal systems and our bodies' ability to lose weight.

Hormones help regulate our weight because they can trigger the body to burn calories from either stored body fat, lean muscle tissue, or from the foods recently eaten. When your hormones are out of balance due to stress, you may be fighting a losing battle when it comes to weight loss. Constant everyday stress could trigger hormones that may override any benefits derived from a good diet and exercise routine. Stress plays a key in regulating your hormones. Are you always under lots of stress? Is your life constantly on the go? Are there other health complaints stressing your body? Do you even know where your stress is coming from? How can you tell if stress is affecting your health? Have you been failing with your weight loss goals even though you have been dieting and exercising? These are all questions you may need to answer in order to succeed in a healthy weight loss program. Maybe all the stress you have been living under has thrown your hormones so out of balance that it has contributed to your inability to lose the extra weight and keep the weight off.

9

Secondly, we will discuss the effects foods (diet) have on your blood sugar and how they trigger certain hormonal responses. Is what you eat and drink triggering your body to burn calories from stored body fat, lean muscle tissue, or from what you just ate a few hours ago? Does your diet throw your hormones further out of balance? Can hormonal imbalances cause your body to burn more calories from carbohydrates and proteins instead of from stored body fat? Which foods are you eating? Are you choosing foods that throw your hormones further out of balance? We will explain how certain foods will trigger your body to burn more calories from fat, while other foods will trigger your body to store all those extra calories. Remember, just because you're burning calories doesn't mean you're burning calories from fat.

The final part of this book covers exercise and the type of exercise routine to follow if you want to keep burning calories from fat. We will discuss how to maximize your exercise routine in order to firm and tone the body. Are you exercising? Are you over-training? Do your workouts give you the results you want? Do your workouts trigger your body to burn calories from stored body fat or do you just burn calories? Do you train at an intensity level that is too high and counterproductive?

There are too many Americans who are overweight and not losing weight even though they are cutting calories, fats, and doing some type of exercise. Maybe our hormones and the triggering effects they play on our body due to stress, diet, and exercise need to be examined. Therefore, if you haven't received the results you wanted from all your time, energy, and efforts in trying to lose weight and tone up, this book will help you examine some different questions for this very puzzling issue.

Good Health Versus Good Fitness

Is good health the same as good fitness? Let's spend a moment addressing "good fitness" and "good health." Most people believe if you are in good physical shape then you are in good health. That's not completely accurate! Are you in good physical shape? Are you physically fit? Can you run two miles? Can you do a dozen pushups? Can you hold your breath for a minute? Can you bend over and touch your toes? These are all questions that pertain to good fitness. If you answered yes to all of these questions, you probably are physically fit.

When it comes to good health, however, you should be asking some different questions, such as, how is your cardiovascular system functioning? How are your reproductive, respiratory, nervous, and immune systems functioning? Do you complain of constant fatigue, headaches, depression, and heartburn? Do you suffer from constipation, bloating, and gas? Are you bothered with arthritis, allergies, diabetes, and osteoporosis? These are questions that pertain to good health. If you answered yes to some of these questions, I don't think you can say you are experiencing good health.

As you can plainly see, good fitness is quite different from good health. Let's not assume just because someone looks physically fit from the outside that they are also healthy on the inside. Many men and women with beautiful physiques on the outside may be plagued with fatigue, headaches, digestive difficulties, arthritis, difficulty sleeping, and food cravings on the inside. I believe good fitness begins with good health.

Good health is not merely absence of disease. A better definition of good health should include the words "vigor and vitality for life." Just because you are not diagnosed with some major type of malady such as arthritis, diabetes, osteoporosis, MS, Lupus, Crohn's, or cancer doesn't mean you are in good health. There have been a number of patients I have helped with weight loss who have thought they were in perfect health except for a few extra pounds. However, as we began our consultation we both learned their bodies were giving us many signals (symptoms) that needed to be addressed.

The main point I am trying to make about losing weight and getting healthy is that there could be a Catch-22. We know if we lose weight we become healthier, but for some of us who simply can't lose weight, even though we are dieting properly, it could be a signal that our overall health needs improving first, in order to successfully shed those unwanted pounds. Think about it, if you're dieting well and still unable to drop those extra pounds, that should be a hint that your body isn't being regulated properly. It's out of balance; something is interfering with your body's ability to run smoothly. It may be smarter to not only concern ourselves with losing weight, but also to put a major emphasis on addressing many of the other signals (symptoms) our bodies are giving us.

Patient Story

Debra wanted me to help her with some of her aches and pains as she prepared for an upcoming sports competition. Debra was in excellent physical shape on the outside. Her body fat was about 12% and she worked out 4–6 times a week with both aerobic and anaerobic training.

As we began evaluating her symptoms, we discovered that she suffered from bloating, gas, constipation, sinusitis, difficulty sleeping, migraine headaches, and an inability to stay awake past nine o'clock at night.

Although Debra looks wonderful on the outside, on the inside her body is dealing with various health issues that are hindering her well-being. Therefore, just because someone looks great physically on the outside, don't assume they are also in great health.

In short, "good fitness" does not always equal "good health." I want to bring these two categories closer together, and as we go through this book and follow the Action Steps at the end of each chapter, we should be able to lose that extra weight, while at the same time become healthier.

Summary

- The body burns calories from fats, carbohydrates, or proteins.
- Hormones have a direct response on which calories the body burns for energy.
- The goal of a good weight loss program is to trigger the breakdown of calories from fat.
- Just because you burned 300 calories from exercise doesn't mean you burned 300 calories from fat.
- Stress, diet and exercise trigger various hormonal responses that we have some control over.
- Good fitness is not the same as good health.
- If proper diet and exercise are not promoting weight loss, it may be the stress level in your life that needs some adjusting.

Action Steps

- Finish reading the book and understand the concepts.
- Set a goal for how much weight you would like to lose, what clothes size you want to fit in, or what kind of shape you want your body to become.
- Figure out how long it will take you to reach your goal (how many months or years). Be realistic.
- Write down your goals and look at them every day to remind yourself where you want to be.
- Commit yourself to take the actions needed to achieve your goal.
- Ask a friend or family member to help hold you accountable to your goal.

Chapter Two

Stress and the Adrenal Glands

Let's first discuss stress and how stress affects your body's ability to burn calories from stored body fat. The reason we want to discuss stress is because stress is everywhere and has a direct bearing on our weight loss efforts. We constantly hear how stress affects our health. The more stress we continually place on our bodies, the weaker the immune system becomes.

Stress and the immune system are inversely related. As the stress in your life increases, your immune system decreases. We've heard the stories of people working long hours, not getting enough sleep, eating poorly, etc. These are the ones who very often catch a cold or infection. They overtaxed their immune systems with stress and allowed their bodies to become susceptible to any invading germ, infection, virus, or bacteria.

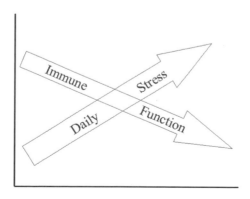

As our stress increases, our immune system decreases.

The immune system keeps you healthy and protects you from infections, diseases, and illnesses. Yet, stress and the amount of stress you place upon yourself can have a direct effect on how successful you are in any type of weight loss program. In fact, excessive, constant stress will begin to exhaust the function of your adrenal glands, which can hinder any weight loss program.

The Adrenal Glands

The adrenal glands sit on top of our kidneys and produce many different hormones that help regulate our bodies. In fact, if the adrenal glands were removed, you would not be able to survive, because they regulate so many different body functions that your body would shut down and die. They are extremely valuable and you never hear of someone having their adrenal glands removed. Most of us may be familiar with the hormone adrenaline and the impact it has on the body. We've heard people speak of an adrenaline rush and that supercharged feeling you get when your body produces extra adrenaline, but there are other hormones produced by our adrenal glands besides adrenaline. Our sex hormones (estrogen, progesterone, and testosterone) are produced by the adrenal glands. They also produce hormones that regulate water, fluids, sodium, and potassium.

Another important feature that is overlooked when examining the function of the adrenal glands is that they help regulate our blood sugar. This can be very important if you are trying to lose weight or if you always feel hungry, light-headed, and irritable if you go more than a few hours without eating, because regulating your blood sugar is crucial in a successful weight loss program.

One of the main responsibilities of the adrenal glands is to produce hormones that respond to stress. Many people overlook the effects of stress and the importance it plays in our weight loss efforts. However, when you're under constant stress, the adrenal glands produce hormones in response to that stress to protect our bodies from whatever stress may be attacking. When the adrenal glands are constantly being required to respond to stress they can eventually reach a point where they become exhausted or depleted. When that occurs, your body's ability to burn calories from fats will diminish. The most important aspect you need to achieve to succeed in maintaining a healthy weight loss program is getting your body to burn calories from stored body fat. However, when your adrenal glands are exhausted and fatigued due to constant everyday stress, this causes an over- or under-production of various hormones that can trigger the body to burn calories from proteins (lean muscle tissue) and carbohydrates instead of stored body fat.

Knowing that, ask yourself: how is the stress level in your life? Is the stress high enough that it keeps driving your hormones further out of balance? Can the hormonal imbalance caused by the constant stress in your daily life be triggering your body to store more body fat than it can burn?

Many patients complain that their thyroids are under-active and that is the reason they can't lose weight and keep it off. However, it is possible the adrenal glands are depleted and exhausted due to constant stress that is slowing down or interfering with the function of the thyroid. This can explain why so often patients who suspect or complain of an under-active thyroid can notice great improvement when they begin nourishing their adrenal glands and thyroids together.

Patient Story

Sue was having difficulty losing weight. She had previously been told her thyroid was the problem and had been taking medication and nutritional supplementation to support her thyroid.

As I was evaluating Sue, she told me that the mental stress in her life is constant and doesn't seem to be getting any better. Many of her symptoms (fatigue, weight gain, poor digestion, constipation, irritability if meals are delayed or missed, mid-afternoon cravings, low blood sugar and the need to eat every 2–3 hours) made me suspect possible adrenal exhaustion.

After identifying some of the things she was doing that were interfering with her health, I implemented a plan that was designed to reduce some of those symptoms and properly support her adrenal glands. Within a few short weeks, her list of health complaints were diminishing and she finally started losing those inches that before seemed impossible for her to lose.

The constant stress placed on the adrenal glands can create hormonal imbalance, which could be affecting your thyroid. This sets up a domino effect. The exhausted adrenals can affect the function of the thyroid, which affects how fast we burn calories. This can cause food cravings that can lead to poor choices of food selection, which can lead to nutritional deficiencies that could lead to having a weakened immune system that allows for the susceptibility to infections and illness, and so on and so forth. It's like a vicious cycle. One hormone out of balance can trigger a whole host of other reactions and imbalances that may have a negative effect on your body and your health.

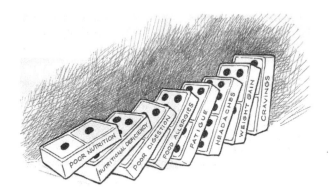

Remember, the thyroid regulates the rate at which the body burns calories in our little fireplace, not so much where those calories are coming from. We burn calories from fats, proteins, and carbohydrates. Our goal should be to make sure the body is in a constant state of burning calories from fat, specifically fat stored on the body. **However excessive, constant stress will prevent the body from being able to burn calories from fats.** The constant daily stress you place on yourself may be what is triggering your body to only burn calories from carbohydrates and proteins and not calories from stored body fat. This is why controlling stress is such an important piece of the puzzle in our efforts to succeed with any healthy weight loss program.

Where Does Stress Come From?

We have all heard the expression "the straw that broke the camel's back." How does that statement apply to you? For most, it simply means that if you continue to pile more and more stress (straws) on your body each day, that load will become so heavy it will

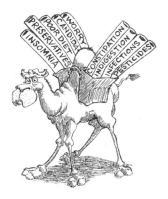

How many straws are you carrying around each day?

eventually break your camel's back. Ask yourself which straws you are constantly carrying each day that are causing your camel to work harder. The point is, if you reduce some of the straws from your camel's back, he'll be able to carry the load much more easily. This is so important because there will be times in your life when you'll have to carry additional straws, and if your camel is already overloaded it will break his back. This is how disease and dysfunction begins to tear away at your health.

The human body is very similar to the analogy of the camel. If you continue to keep adding more stress onto your body, it will catch up and eventually affect the function of your health unless you learn to limit or reduce the stress in your life. **As stress increases, your immunity decreases.**

The body is capable of responding to huge amounts of stress; however, constant stress that lasts for days, weeks, months, years, and decades affects your immune system and eventually wears down the functional capabilities of your adrenal glands.

Think of the adrenal glands as a thoroughbred horse. This horse can run strong and hard when needed. However, this thoroughbred horse also needs to be properly **rested** and **nourished**. How good of a job do you do in resting and nourishing your adrenal glands? Is the stress in your life so high that it is making your horse run hard every day? Are you making your horse carry a heavy load of straws (stress) strapped to its back? Don't you realize if you take some of the weight off its back, it will run better? You cannot expect your horse to run like a champion if you make it run hard every day. That horse needs to be rested and nourished, just as you do. If you want your body to be able to handle all the stress you place on it each day, make sure you are resting and nourishing your body, as well as reducing the amount of stress you place on yourself each day.

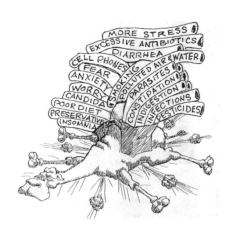

Have you over-stressed your camel?

When patients complain of fatigue, depression, inability to concentrate, weight gain, PMS, irritability, food cravings, and other uncomfortable symptoms, I usually begin with a variety of questions, such as: How's the stress in your life? Do you complain of bloating, gas, or indigestion? How are you nourishing your body? Do you exercise? Are you resting your body? You can't expect your body to operate like a champion if you keep adding more stress to your life.

Patient Story

Robyn came to my office wondering why she hadn't been able to lose weight even though she claimed to be faithfully following a diet and exercise program. She had gained 35 pounds over the last four years and had tried everything to lose the unwanted weight. She was always on the go from morning until nighttime and said her stress level always seemed to be mounting.

After evaluating her list of symptoms, which included fatigue, low blood sugar, mood swings, sweets craving in the afternoon, caffeine to keep going throughout the day, lightheadedness, difficulty with her monthly cycle, allergies, two rounds of antibiotics the past year, history of yeast infections, constipation, bloating, and gas, she realized that her health was not as good as she thought.

We implemented a plan to repair her digestive system, which ensured better absorption of the nutrients that were specifically targeted for her adrenal glands. Within a couple of weeks she started feeling less fatigued, her food cravings diminished, the bloating and gas were gone, and her allergies lessened. After only a month's time of nourishing her adrenal glands, she lost 10 pounds and finally slid below 160 pounds, which she hadn't been able to do for two years.

It was an accumulation of all the different types of stress that was over-taxing her body and triggering all the wrong hormones. Her body was constantly burning calories from carbohydrates and proteins, not stored body fat, due to all the stress that was attacking her body.

As we have covered, the adrenal glands respond to stress, and if the adrenals are exhausted, not only will you have a difficult time losing weight, but you may also suffer from fatigue, low blood sugar, food cravings, allergies, PMS, menopause, asthma, depression, high blood pressure, headaches, irritability, mood swings, digestive difficulties, inability to concentrate, anxiety, and difficulty sleeping. If this sounds like you, then you need to do a better job of resting your body, but also specifically nourish your adrenal glands and look to see where all your stress is coming from.

I think it's important to look at stress and your immune system from two opposite sides of a teeter-totter. First, you need to lower the amount of stress you tax your body with, and secondly, increase and strengthen your adrenals and immune system with proper nutrition.

One of the main functions of the adrenal glands is to produce hormones in response to stress. The over- or under-production of these hormones can be measured to determine the level of stress we are under. This is very useful information to determine the functional capacity of our adrenal glands and our immune function. This may provide the answers to our inability to lose weight, but also why many other health complaints are affecting us.

We will discuss later how to measure adrenal stress, but let's first review the different types of stress, because most people believe there is only one type of stress—mental and emotional stress. Unfortunately, there are several other forms of stress that we need to be aware of and include in our self-evaluation of the amount of stress we tax our bodies with.

Types of Stress

Mental/Emotional Stress—worry, anger, frustration, fear, depression, anxiety.

Physical—obesity, too much exercise, not enough exercise, inadequate or poor sleep, repetitive physical stress, injuries, accidents, trauma, aches and pains, surgery.

Chemical—prescription drugs, over-the-counter medications, pesticides and insecticides in our food, antibiotics, processed and refined foods, artificial sweeteners, colors, flavors and preservatives, toxic or heavy metal exposure, polluted air and water.

Internal Pollution—constipation, diarrhea, indigestion, heartburn, bloating, gas, acid reflux, food allergies, irritable bowel syndrome, leaky gut syndrome.

Microbial Toxicity—overgrowth of candida, yeast, fungus, and parasites.

Nutritional Deficiencies—inadequate supply of vitamins, minerals, antioxidants, essential fatty acids, enzymes, and fiber.

Electro-Magnetic—constant exposure to electro-magnetic waves from computers, televisions, cell phones, microwaves, fluorescent lights, electric blankets, waterbeds, pagers, hair dryers, and clock radios.

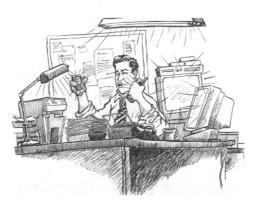

How much electro-magnetic stress are you exposed to each day?

The IRS Approach to Functional Healing
I = Identify & Implement
R = Remove & Repair
S = Support & Strengthen

As you can see, there are many different types of stress that affect our health that we oftentimes don't think about. The IRS Approach to Functional Healing is both an acronym and a process your body moves through as you restore your health. It is a step-by-step process that helps each person know where they are in the healing process as they work toward better health. It is often overlooked, but the more you tax your body with different types of stress, the harder your immune system has to work. As in real life, the greater the tax, the greater the burden. Are you over-taxing your body? Are you making your adrenal glands work too hard? If you are, this could have a big effect on your body's ability to burn calories from fat.

Looking at the different types of stresses in your life you may realize that you may be placing too many straws on your camel's back, which may be the cause of your inability to lose weight. As I said earlier, you cannot only look at someone's desired weight loss goals and design a plan without taking into consideration all the different symptoms that are affecting their health. All those symptoms such as: headaches, fatigue, bloating, PMS, cravings, low blood sugar, irritability, etc. are communicating something to us. Whether we want to take the time and listen to what our bodies are trying to say is the question that needs to be answered. Our bodies are letting us know that something isn't working right, and there's some imbalance that is causing all those symptoms.

If your goal is to successfully lose weight and keep it off, it is important to first get healthy. The IRS Approach to Functional Healing is designed to restore health, which will improve your weight loss results. The first part of the IRS Approach to Functional Healing is to *Identify* all the different stresses that are taxing your body and interfering with your body's natural innate ability to heal itself, then *Implement* a plan that can be followed that will begin to restore health.

The second phase is to *Remove* any toxins, microbes, and any other harmful waste products that are known to interfere with our health and cause dysfunction and disease. Once that has been completed, you can begin to *Repair* any organ or body system that has been affected by the additional stress.

The final part of the IRS Approach to Functional Healing is meant to *Support and Strengthen* the body with proper nutrition and supplementation. It surprises me how many patients are taking twenty, thirty, even forty bottles of different supplements and are not feeling great. I'm a big believer that repairing someone's health is like painting a house. A good painter knows that before you start slapping paint on the walls, it's smart to prep the walls in order for the paint to stick.

The human body is very similar. There are so many patients who complain of leaky gut syndrome, irritable bowels, heartburn, bloating, gas, indigestion, food allergies, yeast, candida, parasites, constipation, and diarrhea that it affects their ability to absorb nutrients from their food and supplements. These people definitely need to repair their gastrointestinal systems (GI tract) first, in order to promote better absorption of their nutrients; otherwise they may not be getting much value from their supplements. It is often stated, *"You are what you eat."* I think it is more accurate to say, *"You are what your body absorbs and what it doesn't eliminate."* Just because you ate a healthy meal, don't think that you automatically absorbed all the nutrients from that food, especially if you are suffering from some of the symptoms above.

When you are following the IRS Approach to Functional Healing, the goal is a step-by-step process designed to get you healthy and keep you healthy by first lowering the load from all the different stresses that are over-taxing your body. As you do this you will begin to notice the changes in your health and realize that good fitness begins with good health.

Take a look at all the different types of *mental, emotional stresses* that affect your health and your quality of life. If those stresses are high, you need to take some action and lower those stresses. There are many different ways to help you control emotional and mental stress. Whether it is the guidance of a professional counselor, prayer, meditation, biofeedback, hypnosis, or visualization, something needs to be done to lower that tax on your body. The simplest and least expensive remedy you can do to help yourself is to breathe. Slow, deep breathing for a few minutes can dramatically reduce the level of cortisol, a hormone produced by the adrenal glands in response to stress. If you only take five minutes a day to close your eyes and relax for a moment with some deep breathing, you can lower the output of cortisol, which is usually very high when you are stressed. Studies are showing that cortisol can be returned to normal values after twenty minutes of quiet, deep breathing. I think this explains why prayer, meditation, visualization, or any other type of quiet, restful, relaxing technique can be very helpful; it lowers our cortisol levels. We will learn later the effects of cortisol and weight loss.

We all know that fear, anger, and worry contribute to mental stress, but did you know that physical exercise can be stressful? Are you over-training? Do you get enough sleep, enough water? Do you have constant aches and pains that are physically demanding on the body? Are you overweight and physically taxing your joints and bones by carrying around an additional twenty, thirty, or fifty pounds? These are questions to help you determine if you are over-taxing your body with physical stress. Review the different types of *physical stresses that can be affecting* your body and make the necessary adjustment to lower that stress.

Have you thought about all the different *chemical stresses* you put in your body? Drugs and over-the-counter medications can tax our livers, kidneys, and stomachs and affect their functional capabilities. Is the air and water you consume loaded with toxins? Does your diet consist of a lot of processed foods, artificial chemicals, and preservatives, which chemically tax your body? Is the food you eat organic and free of insecticides, pesticides, and antibiotics, or do you consume foods loaded with these chemicals, which further tax our body with unnatural substances? These are some of the chemical stresses we place on our bodies that many people fail to think about when they start wondering why they have a particular health issue. *A good cleansing and detoxification program to remove many of the toxins* that build up in the liver, intestines, kidneys, and lymphatic system can reduce the toxic burden on the body. This is a great starting point for many people who want to become healthy.

Internal stress is something that is often overlooked. When your body is dealing with constipation, diarrhea, leaky gut, irritable bowel, bloating, gas, heartburn, indigestion, and food allergies it is an additional tax on your body. The internal poisoning from constipation is taxing your body. The internal environment your tissues and cells live in can be very toxic. I know I don't want to live in an area where the air pollution is bad, so why would I want to have all my tissues and cells living in a polluted internal environment? It's very taxing! There's a tax to pay for all the bloating, gas, indigestion, and reflux we expose our bodies to. Remember, all those antacids and other medications for bloating, gas, indigestion, and reflux are only Band-Aiding the symptom. They are not treating the cause. *Digestive enzymes, hydrochloric acid, and proper food combining can help relieve internal stress.*

Microbial toxicity is another overlooked stressor. Candida, yeast overgrowth, and parasites are an ever-increasing problem and the cause of many health-related problems. A weakened immune system allows the exacerbation of these problems. One reason why intestinal health is so vital is that over 50 percent of our immune system is found in the digestive system. Internal poisoning can contribute to these problems. Good intestinal bacteria keeps the proliferation of candida and yeast overgrowth to a minimum, but the use of birth control pills, antibiotics, and steroid hormones will contribute to candida and yeast overgrowth. Traveling to a third world country is not the only way to become infected with parasites. Raw foods, pork, sushi, and contaminated food and water contribute to the problem. *Good intestinal bacteria, referred to as probiotics, such as* lactobacillus acidophilus *and* bifodobacterium bifidum, *along with a candida and parasite cleanse, can help reduce microbial stress.*

Nutritional deficiencies can be a major stress that is easily over looked. We can't expect our bodies to function well if we don't give them enough water. How do we expect our bodies to function properly if we don't give the body enough vitamins, minerals, antioxidants, essential fatty acids, and fiber, which are some of the raw materials needed to produce hormones, antibodies, enzymes, and neurotransmitters (brain messengers)? Our bodies don't magically manufacture these things, nor do we have an endless supply that can be manufactured. Therefore, if your body is nutritionally deficient of these nutrients, that is another tax on the body. *A multivitamin/mineral supplement with antioxidants and essential fatty acids will help support and strengthen your immune system.*

Electro-magnetic stress caused by the high-tech world we live in is a newer way of taxing our bodies, which we are only starting to learn about. Computers, cell phones, pagers, televisions, microwaves, and other electrical appliances emit an electromagnetic field. It's important to realize that our nervous systems also use electrical impulses to send information to every muscle, organ, and tissue of the body. It is possible that the electrical magnetic fields coming from these electrical units are interfering with the electrical impulses our nervous systems are transmitting. This could be a reason for some of our health problems and an answer for many people who have not been able to find the answer to their health problems!

We need to remember the earth has a magnetic pull, which is why compasses work. However, when you are inside a building or home with three feet of concrete, insulated walls, and you are bombarded with electro-magnetic energy from computers, cell phones, beepers, microwaves, electrical appliances, televisions, radios, fluorescent lights, etc., this may interfere with that compass. Our nervous systems, just like the compass, may be interfered with as they try to communicate with their organs, muscles, and tissues. *Carrying a bipolar magnet with you during the day as you work around these electro-magnetic fields can help alleviate this tax to your body.* It appears that the magnet works like a bulletproof vest toward EMF. Many of my patients who are required to work around computers, televisions, cell phones, and other electrical appliances have benefited from carrying a bipolar magnet.

As you can see, there are other types of stress besides mental and emotional stress we need to be concerned with. Evaluate each of these categories and identify which of the other types of stress you are burdening your body with. You may find that your emotional stress is in control but you are overtaxing yourself with excessive internal, microbial, and electro-magnetic stress! Or quite possibly, excessive physical and chemical stress along with nutritional deficiencies could be the root cause of your unexplained symptoms or health issues. Does your diet adequately supply nutrients in order to support the function of your adrenals, thyroid, liver, kidneys, brain, heart, etc.? Are you constantly exposing your body to electro-magnetic stress? Are you adding more physical stress to the ledger by working out too hard or too long? If you neglect to recognize some of the other types of stress besides mental stress that can be affecting your health, you may find yourself continually fighting a never-ending battle with a particular health issue. This is why just as in war, if you don't know who your enemies are, you don't know who to protect yourself from. Check to see which stresses in your

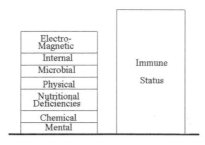

**Cumulative stress greater than immune function.
Highly susceptible to diseases and infections.**

**Immune function greater than cumulative stress.
Highly resistant to diseases and infections.**

life are over-taxing your body. Whatever type of stress is taxing your body, it is important to realize stress has a cumulative effect on your health. Just like the straws on a camel's back, you need to make sure that you are not overtaxing your body with excessive stress, as this weakens your immune system and causes your adrenal glands to work harder. If you keep making your adrenal glands work hard every day because of excessive, constant stress, you eventually exhaust their functional capabilities.

Remember, my underlying goal for this book is to get you healthier while helping you lose weight and keep it off. Identifying where the stress in your life is coming from is the first step needed to promote good health and restore your adrenal glands to proper function. You will see, as you get healthier, the body doesn't need to carry around that unhealthy and unwanted extra layer of fat.

The following is a list of some of the symptoms that are associated with adrenal exhaustion. You may find some of the symptoms that have plagued you could be associated with adrenal exhaustion. This is why it is so important to look at all the different forms of stress that can be overtaxing your body, because all those symptoms can affect the success of your weight loss goals and your overall good health.

Symptoms Associated with Adrenal Exhaustion

• Weight gain or inability to lose weight
• Fatigue and weakness
• Sweets or coffee cravings
• Low blood sugar problems
• Irritable before meals or if meals are delayed
• Shaky or lightheaded if meals are delayed
• Depression, mood swings, irritability
• Difficulty building muscle
• Increased susceptibility to colds, flu, and infections
• Difficulty sleeping or insomnia
• Inability to concentrate
• Premenstrual tension
• Indigestion and poor absorption

- Low body temperature
- Can't fall back to sleep at night
- Reduced immune function
- Poor memory
- Nervousness
- Unexplained hair loss
- Headaches
- Dizziness that occurs after standing
- Anxiety and restlessness
- Palpitations or heart fluttering
- Food or airborne allergies

Do any of these sound familiar or are common symptoms for you? After looking at some of the symptoms associated with adrenal exhaustion, it is important to understand how your adrenals deal with stress.

Summary

- As stress increases, immune function decreases.
- The adrenal glands respond to stress.
- Constant stress can exhaust the adrenal glands.
- Stress can show up as various symptoms.
- Excessive stress can prevent the breakdown of fats.
- There are different types of stress that affect the body.
- Mental/emotional stress.
- Physical stress.
- Chemical stress.
- Internal stress.
- Microbial stress.
- Nutritional deficiencies.
- Electro-magnetic fields.

Action Steps

- Evaluate the different types of stress affecting your health.
- Reduce the stress from each one of the different categories.
- Seek help and advice if you're not sure how to control or manage the stress.

Chapter Three

Stressed about Weight Loss and Fitness

If you had thought that stress only came in the form of mental or emotional stress, the last chapter may have surprised a lot of people. When you think about all the different types of stress that affect your body, is it any surprise to find out that about 75% of all doctor visits are stress related? What we want to talk about now is how the body deals with stress, and what effect does stress have on your body's ability to burn calories from stored body fat?

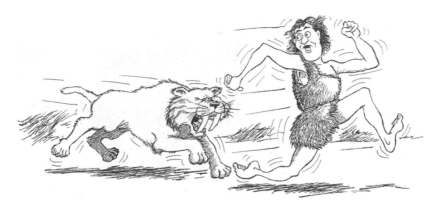

Are you always running from a saber-toothed tiger?

Fight or Flight Versus Resting/Digesting

To better understand what happens to your hormones when you are under stress, you first need to know there are two different systems that constantly regulate your body. The first system is called the

Sympathetic or Fight or Flight Mode. The other is called the Parasympathetic or Resting/Digesting Mode. They are part of the Autonomic Nervous System, which regulates the activities of our breathing, heart rate, blood flow, production of hormones, enzymes, and the activity of our organs. They accomplish this task 24 hours a day, seven days a week automatically, without us ever having to concern ourselves with this process. These two systems can be thought of as opposites, meaning one system turns on or initiates a certain response, while the other system turns that response off or causes the opposite action.

The best way to describe how the adrenal glands respond to stress is the story of coming face-to-face with the proverbial saber-toothed tiger. There are two choices: either run or fight. Neither choice is good, but that is beside the point. The body begins to produce various stress hormones (cortisol, adrenaline, and noradrenaline) to protect itself. These hormones are produced in response to stress, which triggers the beginning of the Fight or Flight mode. Now, you either run or fight to protect yourself, and it is that adrenaline rush you oftentimes hear about that makes you stronger and faster to deal with this situation.

A simple explanation of what happens when the Fight or Flight mode is active is that the body directs more blood to your muscles so you will be strong enough to run away or fight the tiger. The heart rate increases in order to push more blood and oxygen to the muscles. The lungs expand so breathing becomes easier; the pupils dilate so peripheral vision is increased. Blood will be directed away from the digestive system since you don't need to worry about digesting your meal if you're running from a saber-toothed tiger. Once you are out of danger and the stress decreases, the Fight or Flight mode will turn off and the Resting/Digesting mode takes over.

When the Resting/Digesting mode takes over and you're out of danger or not on the go, the heart doesn't need to beat as fast anymore, breathing is slower and deeper and more relaxed, pupils don't open as large and blood doesn't need to be carried to all your muscles so rapidly. All that energy can now be directed to your digestive system and assist in the process of digesting your food and letting your body recover and repair.

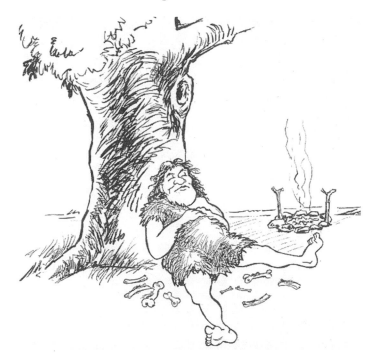

If only every day were like this.

The two systems work in almost direct opposition to one another. When the stress level is high, the Fight or Flight mode turns on several different mechanisms to deal with the stress. Once that stress has been reduced the Resting/Digesting mode will activate and turn off all the switches the Fight or Flight mode turned on. When one system is working, the other one isn't.

The key point I want you to remember is that in a typical day, you should spend most of your time in the Resting/Digesting mode and a short amount of time in the Fight or Flight mode. It's literally impossible to run from the saber-toothed tiger all day long. Unfortunately, many of us do not keep the proper balance of these two systems and spend more time in the Fight or Flight mode. Although you have no conscious control of the different hormonal responses each system triggers, you do have control over which system you spend most of your day in. Are you constantly in the Fight or Flight mode throughout the day? Are you truly in the Resting/Digesting mode when you eat and rest? Do you eat most of your meals on the go? Some people don't know what it is to rest and relax because they are constantly on the go. You need to ask these questions because *when the body is under constant, everyday stress, the stress hormone cortisol is produced, which triggers the breakdown of calories from carbohydrates and protein (muscle), while inhibiting the breakdown of fats.*

Fortunately, we don't have to worry about saber-toothed tigers any longer, but many of us are constantly being chased by what I call "paper tigers." We don't get enough sleep, rush to work in the morning, have a quick breakfast (if at all), rush to feed the kids, hurry to get the kids to school, rush to the office, fight traffic, deadlines, meetings, office politics, quick lunches, road rage, pick up the kids, soccer practice, make dinner, homework, take care of the house, spend time with the spouse, bedtime . . . then start all over again tomorrow. Yet, this is only an example of the mental stress we are under from being on the go all day long. It doesn't include the physical, chemical, internal, microbial, electro-magnetic, and nutritional stresses we tax our bodies with each day.

If this sounds like some part of your day, there is a good chance you are spending too much time in the Fight or Flight mode, which is causing your body to produce more cortisol. The body always feels like it is under attack. We should spend more of our day in the Resting/Digesting mode. Whether you realize it or not, you're creating a hormonal imbalance that will eventually deplete and exhaust the functional capacity of your adrenal glands and their ability to properly respond to stress. A domino effect of dysfunction begins and unexplained symptoms develop that can hinder your health and vitality. This is why it's important to examine the different types of stress that affect your life and adjust your lifestyle so that you are not constantly in this Fight or Flight mode. If you are living a life under constant stress, causing the cortisol levels in your body to be high, this could explain why you have been unable to lose weight, keep it off, and add muscle to your body. You're constantly triggering your body to burn calories from carbohydrates and proteins.

If you remember our analogy about the cabin in the woods and the different types of wood, we only have a limited amount of twigs (carbohydrates) and small branches (protein). If you are constantly complaining of low blood sugar, cravings, light-headedness, irritability if your meals are missed or delayed, and the need to eat every couple of hours, that is a good signal your body is constantly burning up all the carbohydrates.

Early in the book I said that the thyroid regulates our metabolisms, which means it controls how many calories we burn or how hot do we let the fire burn. I also said the adrenal glands help regulate which stack of wood to toss into the fire because we can generate the same amount of heat by either burning lots of twigs and small branches or a few big fat logs. Remember it's more **efficient** to burn those big fat logs rather than to constantly keep adding more and more twigs and small branches into the fire.

Here's the key! If your cortisol levels are constantly elevated due to stress, your body will constantly be forced to burn calories from carbohydrates and proteins. It literally won't be able to burn fats! It's as if someone placed a tarp over the stack of big fat logs we have stored up, and we can't use them to keep the fire going. So just because you're burning calories and have the fire blazing, you need to ask yourself: Does your little fireplace only burn twigs and small branches to keep the fire going? Have you thrown a tarp over the stack of big fat logs you have stockpiled away, making it impossible to burn fats?

The Three Stages of Adrenal Stress

The adrenal glands don't exhaust overnight. It takes time and abuse for this to happen. It was the brilliant researcher, Hans Selye, who first identified the effect stress has on the adrenal glands and their ability to function properly. He coined the term General Adaptive Syndrome and found there are three stages the adrenal glands go through in response to stress.

The first is called the *Alarm Stage.* This is what happens to the body when you see the saber-toothed tiger: heart rate increases, pupils dilate, breathing increases, blood is transported to the muscles and shunted away from the digestive system. All of these activities are turned on and are controlled by the Fight or Flight mode. Once you get out of danger and the stress decreases, the Resting/ Digesting mode will turn off all those body functions that were called into action. The adrenal glands will be able to rest and not have to work and produce cortisol, once you are out of harm's way.

It is in Stage Two and Stage Three that all the problems begin. Stage Two is called the **Resistance** or **Adaptive Stage.** This is when the stress is constant in your life and the adrenal glands are required to produce large amounts of cortisol every day. It's like asking the military to be at the highest level of alert for a long period of time. The body is trying to adapt to this stressful situation. The questions are: How long can your adrenals be expected to produce all these stress hormones before exhaustion and depletion set in? How long before you break your camel's back and symptoms of ill health begin? Remember, your body doesn't have an endless supply of hormones that can be produced at any time! *Your adrenal glands require specific nutrients to help make various hormones.* If your body doesn't have those nutrients or you have depleted the supply of those nutrients, your adrenal glands won't be able to adequately respond to all the stress, and your body will begin to suffer.

The difficulty lies in the fact that you can only be at that constant state of readiness for so long before fatigue and exhaustion set in. That's why Stage Three is called the **Exhaustive Stage.** The body is still under attack from all the constant stress. The only difference is that, because it has been at such a high state of alert for a long period of time, the body, and your adrenal glands, are exhausted and unable to adequately defend themselves from an attack. The prolonged stress has finally caught up and your adrenal glands are unable to respond due to the constant stress. They have been exhausted and are simply worn out and incapable of producing the necessary stress hormones due to excessive stress and inadequate nourishment. When this occurs, dysfunction and ill health begin.

Stage Three, or **Functional Adrenal Exhaustion** as it is referred to, can be likened to the boxer who enters the final round of the fight and needs to keep fighting, but is so fatigued and tired he doesn't have the energy or strength to keep his arms up to fight and defend himself. He is virtually defenseless. That's what functional adrenal exhaustion is like. Our immune (defense) system becomes vulnerable. We want to be able to get up and go throughout the day, after work, and on weekends but we just don't have enough energy to keep going. How many people feel this way? Many people wonder why they are constantly exhausted, tired, fatigued, complaining of food cravings, low blood sugar, irritability, weight gain, PMS, depression, and the list goes on. One common thread of similarity I find with those people who have many of the above-stated complaints is that they are suffering from functional adrenal exhaustion.

Cortisol and Weight Loss

How this applies to weight loss is profound because when you are under continual stress, the body produces a stress hormone called cortisol. Cortisol is very important for maintaining good health, but cortisol triggers the breakdown of carbohydrates and proteins, not fats. Therefore, if you are under a great deal of stress for long periods of time and not getting the results you expect from all your dieting and exercise efforts, you should see how many of the different types of stress you are taxing your body with each day. Are your adrenal glands being triggered to produce a large amount of cortisol every day? Remember there are many different types of stress we need to be aware of. A 24-hour saliva test (we will discuss later) is the best way to measure cortisol levels, which directly reflects the amount of stress your body is under.

When the stress in your life is constantly high or on the rise, this eventually exhausts your adrenal glands and their ability to function properly. This is referred as "hypoadrenia" or "functional adrenal exhaustion." The word "hypo" means low, in this case the low functioning status of the adrenal glands. *If you suffer from hypoadrenia or low functioning adrenal glands, this could explain why you have a difficult time losing weight and adding muscle tone and are always fatigued! Why you are constantly fighting infections and allergies! Why menstrual cycles and menopause are difficult! Why you complain of food cravings, low blood sugar, and digestive prob-*

lems! Why you have mid-afternoon slumps, feel irritable, moody, and depressed! Why you have difficulty sleeping and concentrating!

As you can see, the adrenal glands not only produce our stress hormones, but they are intimately involved in many other aspects of our health. As we said before, we can't keep running from that tiger all day. The adrenal glands are very involved with all these issues and have a domino effect on our health and immune systems. If your adrenal glands are exhausted and overtaxed, so is your immune system. When the immune system is down you become susceptible to all kinds of diseases, infections, and illnesses. This is why it is so important to manage all the different types of stress in your life and properly nourish and rest your adrenal glands. Don't expect your champion racehorse to run every day unless you adequately rest it and properly nourish it each day. If you keep running it every day without the proper rest and nourishment, it'll eventually exhaust. Ask yourself, are you running each day of your life without the proper rest and nourishment to meet your needs? If so, you better think about making some changes in your life before you exhaust yourself and you become defenseless. Remember, good fitness begins with good health.

Many patients, due to our fast, hurry-up society, are suffering from hypoadrenia or adrenal exhaustion. Those who are suffering and not getting better from many of today's health complaints such as fatigue, obesity, food cravings, low blood sugar, depression, PMS, menopause, insomnia, mood swings, irritability, as well as some of the other degenerative and autoimmune diseases, should investigate how well they are controlling the different stresses in their lives. Are you adequately nourishing your adrenal glands for the amount of stress you are placing them under? Have you placed too much stress on your adrenal glands for too long? Are you suffering from hypoadrenia or functional adrenal exhaustion?

Functional Adrenal Exhaustion

Now let's explore what happens when the adrenal glands are in *Stage Two (Resistance)* or *Stage Three (Exhaustion).* When the body is under stress, a hormone called cortisol is produced. The benefits from cortisol are immense. Cortisol works as an anti-inflammatory and helps with the reduction of pain, swelling, and allergic responses. Athletes receive shots of cortisone to help reduce pain or inflammation. Doctors recommend cortisone to help reduce itching and allergies. Cortisol is a beneficial hormone and is involved in many bodily functions. The point you need to understand is that an elevated supply of cortisol running through your body can have some negative effects on your health.

When you are in Stage Two of functional hypoadrenia your body is making more cortisol due to the constant stress. The effects of cortisol are quite simple. It promotes the breakdown of protein (lean muscle tissue) and carbohydrates, which is the last thing we want in any weight loss program. Instead we want to be burning calories from fat. However, the excessive production of cortisol inhibits the breakdown of fat. Therefore, if your body is constantly making more cortisol throughout the day in response to stress, you will have a more difficult time burning body fat and building muscle.

I did not say you would not be able to lose weight! An important issue to understand is that even if you lose weight, you may not necessarily lose body fat. Remember, cortisol promotes the breakdown of protein (lean muscle tissue). Did the weight you lost come from stored body fat, or did you lose lean muscle tissue? Sure, you may have lost 20 pounds in 30 days, but was it body fat? This is one reason I don't like to only use the scale to determine the effectiveness of a weight loss program. I encourage people to use their mirrors and see how their clothes are fitting. Too often patients complain of losing weight, but they are not getting any firmer. Typically, they burn lean muscle tissue, which is why their scales show they lost weight, but their percentage of body fat remains the same. The goal is to trigger the body to burn calories from stored body fat.

Another effect of constant cortisol production is that it can increase the production of acids or decrease the sensitivity to acids in the digestive system. This can lead to ulcers and other digestive difficulties like heartburn, indigestion, bloating, and gas. Excessive cortisol will decrease the production of white blood cells and cause shrinking of our lymph nodes, which causes a decline in our immune systems and allows us to become more susceptible to infections, diseases, and illnesses. Excessive cortisol can promote high blood pressure and other vascular disorders, along with an increase in the breakdown of bone, which can be attributed to osteoporosis.

Stage Three of functional hypoadrenia is when the body can't keep up with the demands that are being placed on it. As we said earlier, you can only go so long with this high level of alert before you deplete and exhaust the functional capacity of the adrenal glands. When this happens, the body can't even make enough cortisol, which is essential for preservation, and we become even more susceptible to other health complaints.

I hope you understand why it is important to examine the different types of stress in your life and see how that can not only affect your weight loss goals, but also your overall health. This is why I emphasize getting the body healthier, not just thinner.

What Hormones Do

We've been speaking about controlling all the different types of stress and how stress can cause an over- or under-production of cortisol. Since the adrenal glands are involved with the production of estrogen, progesterone, testosterone, and DHEA (dehydroepiandrosterone), it's important to see if we are abusing our adrenal glands and upsetting the balance that these hormones have with each other. Hormone imbalances are typically caused by some of the lifestyle choices we make.

Hormones are produced in the body much like anything else, through an assembly line. Let me explain how this assembly line is structured. First, the adrenal glands are responsible for the production of many of the hormones we are familiar with. In fact, cholesterol is the raw material that is used to produce all our hormones. It's unfortunate that we have been led to believe that cholesterol is bad for us because cholesterol is vital for every cell in our bodies. Our adrenal glands will take cholesterol and move along that assembly line to produce a hormone called pregnenolone. Pregnenolone has been referred to as the "mother of all hormones," because without pregnenolone you can't make any of the other hormones.

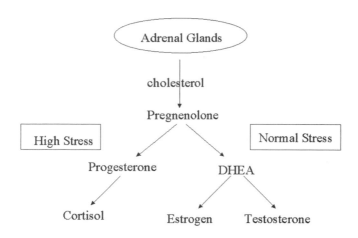

From pregnenolone, there appears to be a "fork in the road," and at this point the assembly line can be directed one of two ways. If there is a lot of stress in your life, your assembly line will be directed to produce progesterone, which is then converted to produce cortisol. Remember, cortisol is produced in response to stress and causes the body to burn calories from carbohydrates and proteins.

If there is not a lot of stress in your life or you are able to properly manage your stress, your body will be able to take its production of various hormones along the other road and produce DHEA. Many of us have heard about DHEA because DHEA has been referred to as the "anti-aging hormone." From DHEA we can then produce estrogen and testosterone, which are very important hormones for both men and women.

DHEA is known to help reduce body fat, increase lean muscle, alleviate depression, strengthen the immune system, increase energy, balance blood sugar, reduce joint pain, promote mental clarity, revitalize our sex lives, and the list goes on. The benefits of the production of DHEA are profound for the body. However, as we age, the production of DHEA decreases, which may explain why it is called the anti-aging hormone. Another feature we are learning is that many people who suffer from various degenerative illnesses and other health-related problems have a lower level of DHEA than someone without the same related health problems.

Now, this doesn't mean you should go and start taking DHEA or pregnenolone for any of your health-related problems, but you need to understand there is a relationship between DHEA and cortisol. If you are constantly asking your body to make more and more cortisol, due to stress, you may eventually get to the point where you are not making an adequate amount of DHEA, which means you don't get to reap all the benefits DHEA provides.

In case you have forgotten, cortisol burns calories from carbohydrates and proteins, while DHEA is known to burn calories from fats, and the name of the game in any weight loss program is not to simply burn calories, but to burn calories from fats! Therefore, controlling the amount of stress in your life can have a tremendous effect on your weight loss program. In fact, you may be following the best diet and exercise program around, but because of all the excessive stress you are under, you may be negating all the benefits from your diet and exercise program.

I am going to veer off of diet for a second and talk about health and the importance of hormonal balance. Ladies, please understand that before menopause your ovaries produce most of your estrogen, progesterone and testosterone. Once you reach menopause or have a hysterectomy you than transfer all the hormone production exclusively to the adrenal glands. Typically that's not a problem, but if you're already overtaxing your adrenal glands, how do you expect them to handle the additional work? This could be the reason so many people have a problem with menopause: their adrenal glands can't take on any more work. This takes us back to the underlying theme of this book—we need to lower or manage the stress in our lives better!

Let's continue. When you lower your stress, you give your body the chance to continue down that hormone assembly line and produce testosterone. Testosterone is important for both men and women because decreased levels of testosterone are associated with both a diminished sex drive and depression. So with so many people complaining of a decreased libido and depression, wouldn't it make sense to start lowering the stress in your life so your body can naturally start producing its own testosterone? Sure, you can go and get an injection of testosterone from your physician to help you with these problems, but you're really not treating the cause of your problems; you're only treating the symptoms. If you go and start adding testosterone to your body, you may be creating a hormonal imbalance that can produce another set of symptoms. Therefore, get back to the basics, "treat the cause—not the symptom," and lower the stress in your life. Remember, "good fitness begins with good health."

Patient Story

Mindy came to my office at the urging of her husband to seek advice for hormonal irregularities and premenstrual syndrome. She complained of always feeling irritable, with huge mood swings and difficult periods that lasted more than seven days. She wasn't able to lose weight even though she followed a regular workout routine. Her job was demanding and stressful, as was keeping up with three teenagers.

She had overwhelmed herself with so much stress that her body was unable to make the necessary hormones to keep up with her busy life. After reviewing her whole history, one of the suggestions I gave her was to begin using progesterone cream topically. She immediately noticed changes. Her energy level improved, her mood stabilized, and her periods became more regular with less cramping.

Being under so much stress, her body was using all that progesterone to make cortisol, which probably didn't leave enough progesterone to produce the other hormones and to keep them in balance. As she supported her body with additional progesterone, her body was better able to make these other hormones, which helped alleviate many of her symptoms.

Measuring Adrenal Exhaustion

There are a couple of simple tests that can be done at home to measure the functional status of the adrenal glands. The first is to take your blood pressure lying down, then immediately take it standing. What should happen is that the systolic (top) number should automatically increase 6–10 points. If it stays the same or falls, that is a good indicator that the adrenals may not be functioning as well as they could. They're not broke, but they're just not doing the job. That is why it is referred to as the "functional hypoadrenia."

Many health professionals assume the adrenals are either broken or they are perfectly fine. I believe there is a "gray area" where they aren't functioning as they should. It's like having two cars traveling from point A to point B. They can both get you there, but one is leaking oil, overheating, and backfiring. You can't assume because they both carried you there they are both working the same.

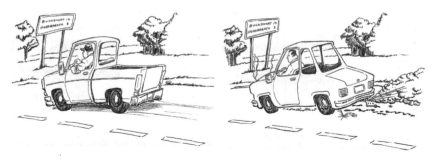

The ride's just not the same in both vehicles.

A second simple test to determine the functional status of the adrenal glands is to take a penlight and shine it into the eye. A normal response is the pupil will constrict and become smaller from the bright light. If the pupil cannot stay constricted and looks as if it is pulsating, this is another signal the adrenal glands may need some attention.

A 24-hour hormonal saliva test is one of the best ways to measure the functional status of the adrenal glands. I recommend a hormonal saliva test to many of my patients who not only have a difficult time with weight loss and fatigue, but also to those patients who may be suffering from various health conditions that don't seem to get any better. A 24-hour saliva test is the best way to measure the production of cortisol and DHEA, which can readily determine the balance of these two hormones and reflect how stress is affecting your health. A saliva test is a better indicator for the functional status of the adrenal glands, because the saliva test is done with four measurements throughout the day as opposed to one measurement that is usually done with a blood analysis. The reason we want to measure the cortisol status for the whole day is that in a 24-hour period the cortisol levels fluctuate. A one-time blood draw won't be able to give as much good information as a 24-hour saliva test will. In addition, the saliva test can be done at home, which eliminates the stress and anxiety of going to the doctor's office, which has been known to cause an abnormal rise in cortisol levels.

If you think your adrenals could be the reason for your lack of success with your weight loss efforts and you have answered yes to many of the questions for the symptoms associated with hypoadrenia, I would seriously examine all the different types of stress that could be affecting not only your weight loss efforts but also your health. So begin to manage and reduce your stress, because it could be the major culprit in your weight loss problems and could be triggering your hormones to constantly burn carbohydrates and proteins for energy and not fat. It's not just burning calories that is important, but it's burning calories from stored body fat that will finally give us the results we want from our weight loss efforts.

Where Does Energy Come From?

For weight loss and dieting purposes, limiting stress and the production of cortisol is crucial. With excessive amounts of cortisol being produced, the liver is unable to break down fats and instead breaks down carbohydrates (sugars) and proteins (lean muscle) for energy. The breakdown of fats is the most efficient way for the body to produce energy. In fact, one gram of fat will produce more than two and a half times more energy than a gram of carbohydrate or protein.

47

To achieve long-term benefits of a healthy weight loss program, it is essential to trigger those hormones that are responsible for the breakdown of fats. When you're always triggering the breakdown of carbohydrates (sugar), it's easier to use up all the sugar in your body, which can explain why 2–3 hours after a meal you're complaining of low blood sugar, cravings, fatigue, irritability, etc. Your body was only burning calories from carbohydrates (sugars).

Supporting the Adrenal Glands

When I started this book, I said, "You can't get the right answers if you don't ask the right questions." Therefore, the difficulty you have been having with your weight loss efforts may have only a small amount to do with your diet and exercise program, but rather a great deal to do with your hormones (adrenals) being out of balance due to stress.

One of the biggest assumptions people make each day is that the body has an endless supply of hormones, enzymes, antibodies, and neurotransmitters (brain messengers). People simply assume the body has an endless supply of these. I want to remind you these hormones, enzymes, antibodies, and neurotransmitters that the body manufactures are what I call "end products." Our organs and glands make these essential end products, but in order to manufacture any end product, we first need to start with raw materials. These raw materials (vitamins, minerals, fatty acids, antioxidants) are what the body uses to manufacture all our hormones, antibodies, enzymes, and brain messengers. Ask yourself: are you giving your body all the raw materials it needs to be healthy, or do you feed it junk food and fast food that has no nutritional value? If you're not nourishing your body with enough good nutrients under normal stress conditions, how do you expect to keep it running properly under stressful conditions?

Science has taught us the functions of the hormones produced by the adrenal glands are far-reaching. That is why it is so important that the hormones produced by the adrenal glands be at the appropriate levels to maintain good health. Some of the nutrients that are known to support and nourish the adrenal glands are vitamin C, the B-vitamins, especially vitamin B-5 (pantothenic acid), zinc, magnesium, licorice root, ginseng, withania, cordyceps, and adrenal glandulars. There should be a small amount of these nutrients found in most of your multivitamins, which should be a staple in everyone's diet. If the levels of the nutrients needed to support the adrenal glands are already low due to constant stress and neglect, you need to further increase the nutrients that are specifically known to support the adrenals. There are some nutrition manufacturers that are aware of the effects of hypoadrenia and that market specific products designed to specifically nourish the adrenal glands. These are a good start to help you begin nourishing your adrenal glands.

The hormones DHEA and pregnenolone are two supplements that are highly effective in supporting the function of the adrenal glands. However, I would not recommend taking DHEA without first taking a 24-hour saliva screen to measure your cortisol and DHEA levels. The reason is if you suspect that your DHEA level is low and begin to supplement your diet with DHEA, when in actuality your hormone levels are normal, then you would be contributing to hormonal imbalance and possibly exacerbating health complaints.

When your adrenals are exhausted and you are unable to produce an adequate amount of DHEA, your health could suffer. This is why it is important to rest and properly nourish your adrenal glands, so your body can produce its own DHEA. However, until you can properly nourish your adrenals it may be a good idea to supplement with DHEA and/or pregnenolone. Imagine pushing your car up a hill all day; DHEA is like a friend who comes and helps you push your car. While your friend is pushing your car, you are sitting inside resting and nourishing your adrenal glands with proper supplementation. You're still getting your car moved from point A to point B (your hormones are regulating your body), but once you've had a chance to rest and nourish your body you will again be strong enough to push your car yourself. Remember, you can't ask your friend to push your car all the time.

If you properly nourish your adrenal glands and decrease the excessive stress in your life, your body will do a better job of keeping those hormones in balance. These hormones will then have a triggering effect on your body's ability to burn fat and not store fat, along with your body's ability to control and regulate many of the other symptoms associated with adrenal exhaustion and depletion.

Summary

- You can't run from the saber-toothed tiger all day.
- If you're always struggling with excessive stress in your life it could be hampering your weight loss results.
- Let your body rest, recuperate, and repair.
- Stress triggers the production of cortisol.
- Cortisol breaks down protein (lean muscle tissue) and inhibits the breakdown of fat.
- Deep breathing and relaxation can lower cortisol production.

Action Steps

- If you're not having success with your weight loss efforts and you feel that your adrenal glands may be exhausted, begin to rest, lower the stress on your body, and specifically nourish your adrenal glands.
- Have your cortisol and DHEA levels checked with a 24-hour saliva test.
- Continue to work at lowering the stress in your life.

Chapter Four

Is the Thyroid to Blame?

At the start of this book I spoke of a little fireplace we all have burning inside. If you can imagine, our thyroid glands function much like that fireplace and they're responsible for keeping the cabin (body) warm.

The thyroid gland, the adrenal glands, the pancreas, and our reproductive organs (ovaries and testes) are merely instruments in the orchestra we call our endocrine system. They are just players in the band, but if one instrument is off key and playing poorly, that could disrupt the beautiful sound we expect to hear.

It is common for most people and doctors to suspect the thyroid as the chief problem when weight loss efforts fail, especially when we think our diet and workouts are being followed correctly. What we want to discuss now is the function of the thyroid and its involvement in a good weight loss program.

We just finished learning how stress affects the hormones produced by the adrenal glands and how they can affect our weight loss results. Keep in mind that one hormonal imbalance can trigger another hormonal imbalance. Maybe the function of the thyroid is being affected by the function of the adrenal glands? Maybe the stress in our lives is causing a domino effect on our thyroids?

Metabolism

One of the primary functions of the thyroid is to regulate our metabolism, which is defined as the rate at which the body burns calories.

Many people complain of having a low thyroid or slow metabolism. The importance of burning calories from stored body fat is the most important part of a healthy weight loss plan. *We can be burning hundreds of calories daily, but if those calories are coming from the breakdown of protein (lean muscle tissue) and carbohydrates rather than fats, then this could explain why we may not be reaching our weight loss goals.* The thyroid may be functioning fine at burning calories. However, it doesn't determine the source where those calories come from. We want to make sure we are burning as many logs (fats) as we can. Just because the exercise machine said you burned 300 calories, it doesn't tell you if you burned those calories from the breakdown of fats, proteins, or carbohydrates.

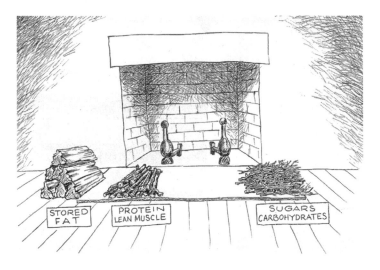

How do you keep your fireplace burning?

Think of the thyroid as a small fireplace responsible for keeping the whole cabin warm. If you place enough logs in that fireplace, it should generate enough heat to warm the whole cabin. However, if you don't place enough logs in the fireplace, you only heat up the area closest to the fireplace and do not generate enough heat to warm the furthest corners of the room. Do you complain of always having cold hands and feet? Maybe your fireplace (thyroid) isn't burning enough logs (calories) to keep the whole room warm. This could be a thyroid problem.

What Is a Calorie?

A calorie is nothing more than a unit of measurement of heat. When you burn a calorie, a certain amount of heat is generated. If your body is burning lots of calories it is generating lots of heat, which keeps the body temperature up. When the thyroid is burning enough calories and generating enough heat, we are usually able to keep the whole body warm, including our hands and feet.

We don't want our fireplace only burning twigs and small branches, we need the fireplace to burn all of the big logs as well, because they give off more heat. This is just like our body, as we don't want to only burn calories from carbohydrates and protein. We need to trigger our body to burn calories from fats, because just like those logs, they give off two and a half times more energy. *Don't assume because you're exercising and burning calories that you're burning calories from fat.* As we already discussed in the previous chapter, our hormones (adrenals) are very involved in determining which logs go into the fireplace.

Basal Metabolic Rate

A great test to determine how well and efficiently your body is burning calories is to measure your metabolism (the rate at which your body burns calories) and get a fix on your basic metabolic rate. Your Basal Metabolic Rate (BMR) is a function of your thyroid and determines the fewest number of calories your body burns to keep you living and breathing. How many calories does your body burn just to live and breathe? We don't want to measure how many calories you burn when you exercise. We want to know how many calories your metabolism is burning at rest. What is your basal metabolic rate? Remember, you only exercise one or two hours a day. The other 22 or 23 hours your body is basically at rest in a resting, digesting mode.

The amount of calories (heat generated) your body burns if you lie in bed all day is considered your basal metabolic rate. Think of your

BMR as the idle speed of your car. If you let the car idle at 1,200 RPM, it will burn gasoline at a certain rate. If you increase that idle speed, by stepping on the accelerator, up to 1,500 RPM, it will burn gasoline at a much faster rate. This is what you want to happen in your body. We need to have our thyroids (metabolism) burning more calories for a successful weight loss program that will help you reach your goals of losing the weight and keeping it off.

Testing the Thyroid

There are two simple tests you can do at home which may give you a clue how your thyroid is functioning. The first test is very simple. You take a tincture iodine, which can be purchased at any local drugstore.

Place a small iodine stain the size of a quarter on the underside of your forearm. If the stain remains for 18–24 hours, it's a good sign your thyroid may not be the problem. However, if the stain disappears and is absorbed within a few hours, that is a clue your thyroid may not be functioning well. Your thyroid may be deficient of iodine and absorbed all it found on your skin. Please realize that placing iodine on your skin is not the best way to nourish your thyroid. Using a supplement would be a better choice.

The second functional test uses a thermometer to measure your body temperature. Dr. Broda Barnes, an endocrinologist, did years of research on thyroid function and found that measuring your underarm (axillary) temperature was a more accurate way of determining body temperature and an excellent way to determine functional status of the thyroid. This simple test will let you know if you are generating enough heat to keep your core body temperature stable. If you are burning an adequate supply of calories your body temperature should be between 97.8 and 98.2 degrees. If your body temperature is below this range, this could be a clue that your thyroid may be underactive.

The most important part of this test is that it needs to be done first thing in the morning before you get out of bed. We are trying to determine your basic metabolic rate (body temperature) before you get up, walk around, eat, and generate any muscle activity. Daily activity will increase your metabolic rate and cause your body temperature to rise. What surprises many patients when doing this underarm test in the middle of the day after indulging in all kinds of activity is that their body temperature is still on the low side. What do you think that tells them? If your body temperature is low in the middle of the day, there is a good chance it is low first thing in the morning and we could be dealing with a thyroid problem.

The second part of this test, besides being done before you get out of bed, is that it needs to be done for at least five days in a row to get a good accurate measurement. Take the average and determine if your body temperature is between 97.8 and 98.2 degrees. The five-day test applies to men and post-menopausal women. If you are still menstruating, I would recommend doing the test for thirty days since some hormones fluctuate during your cycle. Both of these tests are simple, easy to do at home, and are meant to give you an indication as to the functional status of your thyroid.

Revving the Engine

When we begin to trigger our bodies to burn more calories, our chance of successfully losing weight increases. Therefore, the responsibility of the thyroid is to constantly keep that fire burning (our metabolism) as hot as possible. There are four things we can do to increase our metabolism.

First, get some exercise! When we exercise and build muscle we increase our metabolisms. The reason for this is simple: muscle tissue is metabolically more active than adipose (fat) tissue. This means that a pound of muscle burns more calories than a pound of fat. It's as if we are keeping our foot on the accelerator and revving the engine throughout the day when we exercise. So, if you add additional muscle to your body you will be increasing your metabolism. This is why we want to stimulate our muscles and begin some type of daily exercise routine.

Second, eat! When we limit our daily intake of food to one or two meals a day we start slowing down our metabolisms. The body has a survival mode; if it recognizes that it is only getting food (calories), twice a day, it will begin to preserve those calories and burn them more slowly. Therefore, eating only one or two meals a day in hopes of losing weight will cause our metabolisms and thyroids to slow down. Whereas, if you feed your body 3–5 times a day, it stimulates your metabolism to continually burn calories. Therefore, if you're not eating at least three meals a day, it's like swimming upstream. It will be more difficult to lose weight.

Consuming 3–5 meals a day will increase our metabolisms and burn a greater number of calories, but I know eating more than three meals a day is difficult for some people. This is why I encourage people to create a dieting plan they can follow long term. Many patients have told me that they lost weight eating 5–6 meals a day, but found it too demanding to eat that often on a regular basis. In fact, as soon as they went back to eating three meals a day, they regained their weight. Therefore, if you know that you can't eat 5–6 meals a day long-term but can eat three meals, why would you follow that type of dieting plan? Create the habits and dieting plans you can use for a lifetime.

FYI—excess calcium can cause the thyroid and our metabolisms to slow down. It is important to look for a calcium supplement that has magnesium, vitamin D, and boron. Calcium should be consumed at a ratio of no more than two to one with respect to magnesium. If you take 1,000 mg of calcium I suggest you get at least 500 mg. of magnesium. These two minerals are effectively absorbed when taken at a 2:1 ratio. Excess calcium that is not absorbed can begin to calcify and plaque the arteries, which is known as hardening of the arteries. If it doesn't do that, it could begin to calcify in our joints, which can contribute to arthritis. Lastly, it can slow down your metabolism.

Those of you who are swallowing antacids for heartburn, indigestion, bloating, and gas and are combining calcium to help with osteoporosis may not be getting the benefits you think, because an acidic environment is necessary to activate and make calcium, magnesium and other minerals absorbable. Unfortunately, antacids suppress the acidity in the stomach, which interferes with the absorption of these minerals.

Third, various herbal supplements act as thermogenics, which work to heat up the body. The herbs that have been shown to work the best at raising our metabolisms are ma huang and caffeine. Both are classified as stimulants to the body. Therefore, some precaution must be taken when used. These two herbs are commonly found in many of the weight loss supplements that are on the market today. The drawback for many of us who use these supplements for weight loss is that these two herbs, ma huang and caffeine, are known to deplete and further exhaust the adrenal glands. If you are concerned that you have already exhausted your adrenal glands and are working to nourish them, realize these two herbs will be working against you and should be avoided.

As we discussed earlier, when the adrenal glands are in a state of exhaustion, this inhibits the burning of calories from stored body fat. We may burn more calories with these stimulants, but are those calories coming from the breakdown of fats? They may promote the breakdown of proteins (muscle) and carbohydrates due to adrenal exhaustion, which is not what we want in a healthy weight loss program.

A *fourth* solution to help with increasing our metabolisms and BMRs is to look for an underlying problem with the adrenal glands caused by stress. Excess cortisol due to stress will interfere with the production of our thyroid hormones. Think of it like dominos. If the "adrenal domino" falls first, it may knock over and pull down the functional ability of the "thyroid domino." In which case, you need to lift up (support) the "adrenal domino" before you can raise (repair) the "thyroid domino." Many times the exhaustion of the adrenal glands causes a domino effect to our good health. Various health complaints are sometimes the result of another imbalance from within the body. Therefore, the over-production of the stress hormone cortisol, caused by constant excessive stress, could be interfering with the proper function and regulation of the thyroid. This can explain why so many people have an underactive thyroid and are taking medications but not getting the expected results from their medications. Look for a possible underlying adrenal problem, because if you don't fix that first all the medications or supplements that work to raise your metabolism and BMR may be unsuccessful. Look to the adrenal glands first! This is not to say that it couldn't be an actual thyroid problem, in which case we need to strengthen and support the thyroid, which is always a good idea.

Finally, and usually the most important, is to specifically nourish and strengthen the thyroid with good nutrition and proper supplementation. Iodine found in kelp is an excellent source of nourishment for the thyroid. Tyrosine, B-vitamins, selenium, zinc, and thyroid glandulars can also be included in a nutrition protocol to support the thyroid.

Summary

- The thyroid regulates our metabolisms and the rate at which we burn calories.
- A calorie is a unit of heat.
- Increasing our metabolisms promotes the breakdown of additional calories and helps with weight loss.
- Our metabolisms can be increased by:
  — Exercising
  — Eating a minimum of 3–5 meals a day
  — Using herbal thermogenics
  — Nourishing the adrenal glands and thyroid.
- Energy is generated from the breakdown of fats, carbohydrates, and protein.

Action Steps

- Do iodine and axillary temperature tests.
- Begin an exercise program and find ways to stimulate your muscles daily.
- Eat 3–5 meals a day.
- Nourish the thyroid and adrenals if you suspect they need assistance.

Chapter Five

Balancing Blood Sugar

Suppose you had a thousand dollars a month to invest and you could invest in anything you wanted—stocks, bonds, real estate, jewelry, or whatever. One of the most important considerations is the rate of return on your investment. Would you rather invest your hard-earned money in some investment that will give you a return on your investment of 5–10%, or would you rather invest your money in something that would return 40–50% on your investment, the amount of risk being equal?

It's pretty obvious—this is a no-brainer. However, to use the old cliché, "Time is money!" we need to recognize and acknowledge that our time is valuable and whatever time we have to spend on dieting and working out, we should try to optimize our efforts. Are we getting the most out, of the time, energy, and effort we spend each week counting calories, fat grams, watching our diets, and working out?

If you are not getting the results you want, you need to make some changes. There is an old saying that says, "The definition of insanity is doing the same thing over and over again, hoping for a different result." If what you are doing isn't working, then try something else. I said in the beginning of the book that our hormones regulate our bodies and that some hormones burn calories from fats and some hormones burn calories from carbohydrates and proteins. I also said, we have a tremendous amount of control over which hormones we want racing through our body. We've learned which stress hormones burn fats and carbohydrates. Now we are going to learn how diet affects a couple of other hormones that are involved with weight loss.

First, I want to point out the actual benefits we get from both diet and exercise. Roughly 20% of the benefits we receive from exercise come from the actual physical workouts we do; another 20% of the benefits from our workout come from the amount of rest and recuperation we allow our bodies to have, while at least 60% of our benefits from workouts come from our diets. That's right, at least 60% of our benefits will come from our diets!

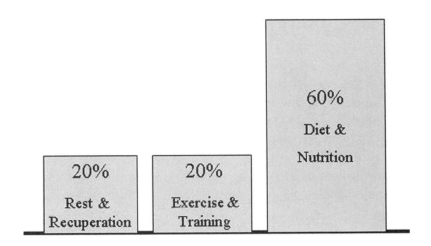

Where do you invest your time, energy, and effort?

With that in mind we need to ask ourselves: in what area are we investing most of our time, energy, and efforts? Are we investing wisely in the area that has the greatest rate of return? Are we investing wisely with our money and poorly with our health? Are the results we get from our workouts as visible as we would like them to be? Perhaps we need to reevaluate and adjust our diets to seek the greatest return for our weight loss efforts.

The Importance of Diet

With at least 60% of the results from our exercise routines coming from our diets, we need to discuss the importance of diet and how to make our diets work for us. First and foremost, when I use the word diet, I do not use it in reference to a restrictive weight loss plan of eating. When I use the word diet, I am simply stating the food and drink we place in our bodies to maintain existence. When we go to the zoo and ask what is the typical diet for the lions, tigers, and bears, we are not thinking they are on some restrictive weight loss program. We are simply trying to determine what lions, tigers and bears eat, not what type of restrictive dieting program they are on.

Let me emphasize that diets in the traditional sense don't work! I want to share with you how the body functions, how our blood sugar controls our hormones, and how we need to control our blood sugar in order to trigger the hormones that will help us burn calories from fats.

First and foremost, when it comes to determining a healthy eating or dieting program, it is of utmost importance to follow a dieting or eating program that is healthy and can easily be maintained for a long period of time. If the dieting program you're following isn't healthy and something you cannot do long-term, you won't succeed. For example, if you follow a restrictive eating program that is difficult to maintain for the long-term or is not nutritionally healthy, you will probably regain the weight. If the dieting plan you're on doesn't promote good health, stay away from it. These are your typical fad diets where you eat or drink certain foods all day long, like shakes, pineapples, watermelons, or grapefruits. Although they may help you lose weight, it may not be weight loss from the breakdown of stored body fat. Furthermore, it may not be nutritionally healthy, meaning it does not supply your body with all the vitamins, minerals, antioxidants, fatty acids, fiber, good bacteria, and other building blocks needed for good health.

Does your weight loss and dieting program emphasize eating 4–6 meals a day, which is more than you have time for in your day? If that is the case, there is a good chance that once you reach your weight loss goal, you may no longer follow a dieting program of 4–6 meals a day, revert back to three meals a day, and regain your weight. Eating 4–6 meals a day does increase your metabolism, but you may be like so many of us in the real world who don't have time to eat 4–6 meals, let alone the time to prepare all those meals. If that's the case, it's important to learn how to trigger your body to burn calories from fats on three meals a day. The reason I say this is because patient compliance and our ability to follow a dieting plan for a long time are major factors for any weight loss program.

Counting Carbohydrates and Fats

Let's bury the myth about fat in our diet. Most people in the last 25 years have been led to believe that fat is bad for our bodies. We have been told that we eat too much fatty food and that this is the leading cause of obesity, heart disease, stroke, and cancer in our society. For the past 25 years we have been eating more calories from carbohydrates and less from fats. While at the same time our rate of obesity, heart disease, stroke, cancer, and diabetes is increasing. Let me clearly state that fat is not the culprit it has been made out to be; it is not bad for us, and is, in fact, essential for our existence. There are some fats that are worse than others, which is why we need to look at different types of fats. There are many cultures that eat more fats than North Americans, yet don't have the same health problems. This is why balancing our fat intake with both monounsaturated and saturated fats is important.

There are three major nutrients we consume each day—carbohydrates, proteins, and fats. Most people know that when we eat carbohydrates, we break the carbohydrates down into sugar and produce energy. Proteins are broken down and used to produce muscle. However, many people believe that the fat we eat has no purpose, except for taste and to make us heavier. In fact, fats are the building blocks for our body to produce hormones.

In the last chapter, we showed how the body uses fats as a raw material to make hormones. If you have been following a low-fat or no-fat diet regimen and not getting the results you have been expecting, and also suffer with PMS, menopause, arthritis, heart disease, or headaches, it may have something to do with the proper amount of fats, specifically the ratio of saturated and monounsaturated fats in your diet. Are we eating enough of the good fats (monounsaturated, omega-3, and omega-6 fatty acids) in our diets? Do we overload our bodies with saturated fats, which when out of balance create many of the health problems our society faces today? We are beginning to learn that many of the abovementioned health problems could be reduced or eliminated when we start to restore the balance of our essential fatty acids (omega-3s and omega-6s) in our diets.

The real problem isn't just the fats in our diets, but rather the excessive sugar (carbohydrates) consumption and what it does to our blood sugar levels! This blood sugar balance is another piece of the puzzle that needs to be intact to achieve long lasting and successful weight loss.

Don't think that I am down on carbohydrates! I am a big believer in the importance and necessity of carbohydrates. Unfortunately, many of today's no-carbohydrate diets are "throwing the baby out with the bath water." I am a big fan of the carbohydrates we get from fruits, vegetables, and whole grains. What I am particularly concerned about is the over-consumption of refined carbohydrates (processed white flour and processed white sugar), which have become a major staple in today's society, and the consequences they have on our bodies' ability to regulate our blood sugar. Since the Garden of Eden until modern times, all the foods we have eaten have been organic and unrefined. The organic food craze was not something that was started by a bunch of hippies back in the '60s out in California. It's been in the last century, with the invention of food processing, that our diets have been drastically disturbed and have changed the ratio of carbohydrates to proteins to fats in our diets. These refined carbohydrates have been triggering our blood sugar levels to skyrocket up and down, which causes hormonal imbalance, which is another piece of the puzzle that needs to be addressed in any weight loss program.

Patient Story

Beverly was a self-admitted carbohydrate junkie who had struggled with her weight for years. She had been eating low-fat and no-fat for years, fearing that fats would make her gain even more weight. Her typical breakfast was a cup of coffee with a bagel or muffin; on others days a bowl of cereal. Lunch was yogurt, rice cakes, crackers, microwave popcorn, or pretzels. She would have a soft drink or cup of coffee to make it through the rest of her day and dinner was usually lots of pasta and breads.

She complained not only of an inability to lose weight but also of low blood sugar, irritability if meals were skipped or delayed, fatigue, light-headedness, PMS, difficulty with her periods, sensitivity to bright lights, and food cravings.

After reviewing her symptoms and diet history, we eliminated refined carbohydrates (foods that are prepackaged with processed white flour and white sugar) from her diet and replaced them with meals that had more protein and good fat. We were trying to stabilize her hormones and not overload the release of insulin. Within a couple of days, her energy level picked up, her cravings subsided, and her need to eat every 2–3 hours was reduced. She wasn't having that drained feeling at mid-afternoon, her periods were less severe, and her weight finally began to drop.

Beverly had been eating so many carbohydrates each day that it was throwing her hormones out of balance and triggering the wrong responses. The body needs carbohydrates; we just need to make sure we don't overload ourselves with too many carbohydrates or the wrong (refined) carbohydrates.

Balancing your blood sugar or keeping your blood sugar from soaring too high or crashing too low is crucial in a successful weight loss program. The goal should be to keep your blood sugar relatively level throughout the day, because when it goes too high or too low it triggers certain hormones to store fat and not burn it. Therefore, if you're having a hard time losing weight and suffer from other health-related complaints, your blood sugar could be at the root of your problems.

Balancing Our Blood Sugar

The two hormones we need to pay close attention to in our quest for losing weight and balancing our blood sugar are *insulin* and *glucagon.* These two hormones are controlled by our diet, and we have control over what makes up our daily diet. What we eat will trigger the release of insulin and glucagon. The role they play is immense and the balance they maintain can make or break our dieting efforts. Most of us are familiar with insulin because of the association it has with diabetes. However, many of us are unfamiliar with glucagon and the role it plays in balancing our blood sugar and promoting the breakdown of fats. These two hormones are inversely related, meaning when one hormone is up, the other is down, and vice-versa. They both work at balancing our blood sugar. Insulin will lower blood sugar, while glucagon will raise our blood sugar.

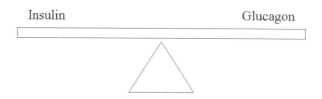

Insulin   Glucagon

A proper diet promotes the availability of both insulin and glucagon.

Insulin is considered an "anabolic" hormone. The definition of anabolic is to grow or to build. The hormone glucagon is considered a "catabolic" hormone, which means to break down or tear apart. If you are trying to lose weight and keep it off, you should be striving to trigger a good balance of both anabolic and catabolic hormones.

The question you need to be asking is: What triggers these responses? Do certain foods trigger the release of one hormone over the other? Do we release enough glucagon to promote the breakdown of fats? Will some foods trigger our bodies to burn fat and other foods to store fat? Your daily food selection can have a huge effect on your hormones and, depending on what you choose to eat, may affect which hormones you produce. Is your diet triggering your hormones to burn or store fat?

If you look at the typical American diet over the last 20 years, it has more or less been a diet of low fat or no fat. In that same time period, we have increased the number of people complaining of heart disease, stroke, diabetes, obesity, high cholesterol, high blood pressure, arthritis, menopause, PMS, etc. We have been led to believe that the problem is fat or excessive fat in our diet. However, if you look at other cultures around the world that eat more fat in their daily diets than Americans do, they do not have the same health complaints —it just doesn't add up!

On paper it looks as though fats could be the problem. A gram of fat is converted into nine calories, while a gram of protein or carbohydrate only produces four calories. When you start adding up and counting how many calories we are ingesting at each meal, we see that calories from fats can really start to add up. This is why for years people have been trying to count calories to lose weight. Who wants to spend all of their time in front of a scale or looking at conversion charts to see how many calories they have eaten?

If we only look at the fat grams or calorie content in our daily meal selections, we are making a mistake. Looking at only fats and calories to determine if we can eat them is like looking at someone's IQ or financial status to determine if you want to be friends with them. We don't pick our friends based solely on these two criteria, nor should we be picking our food based solely on its fat or caloric content.

If it were just fats and calories that were the cause of our high rate of obesity, heart disease, and stroke, then how can we explain the "French Paradox"? It is called the French Paradox because the French eat much more fatty foods than Americans, yet they don't experience the same rate of obesity, heart disease, stroke, diabetes, and other ailments that Americans do. They are eating lots of cheese, sour cream, butter, eggs, and dairy in their diet. Great tasting stuff, but they are all considered no-nos in the American diet. This could help explain why obesity and other health-related problems do not come strictly from too much fat, but instead come from too much sugar (refined carbohydrates) in our daily diet. Americans by and large eat more processed and refined foods, which are loaded with carbohydrates and drive our blood sugar out of balance, than the French.

It is the good fats, the monounsaturated fats (omega-3 and omega-6) that we don't usually eat enough of in our diet to promote good health. The fats that are bad for us are the partially hydrogenated fats or trans fatty acids as they are called. These are the fats that are not beneficial for promoting good health. You can usually find the partially hydrogenated fats in many baked or prepackaged foods. Many of the condiments that we use are loaded with these trans fatty acids. Read your labels. If the ingredient list contains partially hydro-genated fats, try to avoid them as much as possible.

Carbohydrates Do What?

We have been told for the last 25 years to eat no-fat or low-fat foods and eat more carbohydrates. If we don't eat enough good fats (essen-tial fatty acids) due to restricted fat intake, we can be creating an imbalance of all our hormones that are involved in all areas of our lives, not just our reproductive systems. Therefore, if you complain of PMS, menopause, heart disease, arthritis, or headaches and have been on a low- or no-fat diet, I would recommend supplementing your diet with some essential fatty acids (omega-3 and omega-6).

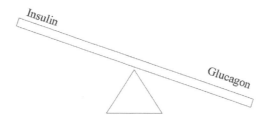

A diet high in carbohydrates causes insulin to increase.

When we eat carbohydrates they are broken down into sugar and released into our bloodstreams. Our blood sugar level increases in response to carbohydrates, which triggers the pancreas to produce insulin. Insulin works to lower our blood sugar by pushing the sugar out of our bloodstream and into the cells, where it can be utilized for energy. This is a beneficial task.

The problem is if the food is heavily loaded with carbohydrates, especially refined, processed carbohydrates, then the blood sugar will elevate quite rapidly and surge very high. If the blood sugar increases rapidly, the pancreas will respond with a huge production of insulin to lower the blood sugar. If our blood sugar skyrockets up, it will then roller coaster down very fast. It is that roller-coaster ride down where many of our problems begin, such as low blood sugar, food cravings, fatigue, irritability, moodiness, light-headedness, and/or irritability if meals are skipped or delayed. Our bodies function much better when we keep our blood sugar fairly level. Those blood sugar surges caused by a diet high in carbohydrates are the real problems behind many of today's health problems along with making it more difficult to lose weight. We have also learned that excessive sugar in our diets heavily taxes our adrenal glands, which is an additional stress that must be dealt with.

Since insulin is considered an anabolic hormone, its effects make us bigger. Not necessarily bigger and stronger, but probably bigger and fatter, if we don't properly control our insulin responses. Insulin also works as a storage hormone and will take the excess carbohydrates and store them as fat.

The breakdown of a meal is relatively simple. Carbohydrates are sugars that are converted into glucose and used for energy. The problem is that we can only utilize so many carbohydrates at each meal. The rest will be stored; some of it will be stored as glycogen, which is a stored form of sugar found in the liver and skeletal muscles. The rest of the carbohydrates are stored as fat.

If you're eating meals loaded with carbohydrates and you're having problems with weight loss, maybe the foods you're eating are triggering a hormonal response that is storing fat and not burning fat.

> *FYI: A high triglyceride count is commonly the result of a diet high in refined carbohydrates. Therefore, decrease the intake of refined carbohydrates and this should help lower your triglyceride count.*

Patient Story

Walter came to me complaining of Type II adult onset diabetes, inability to lose weight, and a high triglyceride count. He was only 33 years of age, somewhat active, but was taking oral medication to control his diabetes and was advised at his last physical that his "HDL" (good cholesterol) was low and his triglycerides were high.

Walter's diet consisted mostly of carbohydrates. Most of his carbohydrates came from refined and processed foods. We immediately reduced his carbohydrates and increased the protein and good fats in his diet. Within a few days, he noticed that his blood sugar had begun to stabilize and his medication needed to be adjusted. Since he wasn't eating so many carbohydrates, he didn't need so much medication to control his insulin. He was feeling better within the first few weeks and a couple of months later he had lost almost twenty pounds. His lab work showed that his triglycerides and good cholesterol were now in normal ranges.

The overload of carbohydrates to his body provoked a domino effect to his health. All of those excess carbohydrates were stored as fat, which created more stress to his heart health.

Here is something to think about the next time you try to load up with a high-carbohydrate meal. What do you think ranchers feed their cattle to get them as fat as possible before they are sold at market? They are fed strictly carbohydrates (grains), which increase their blood sugar and insulin. This overload of insulin triggers the body to convert the excess sugar into fat. Keeping them in pens prevents them from walking around (exercising) and burning off any stored carbohydrates and fats. A great-tasting steak is marbled with fat. Ranchers are not feeding their cattle ice cream and cookies to fatten them up. They are letting them eat more and more grains, which eventually causes hormonal imbalance and makes the cow fatter.

This is the same thing that happens to us when we continually eat a diet high in carbohydrates, especially refined carbohydrates. Maybe that visual will help us turn away from some of the high carbohydrate-rich meals that most Americans eat. These include meal selections such as bagels, muffins, cereals, breads, pancakes, crackers, popcorn, rice cakes, pasta, pretzels, tortilla chips, baked potatoes, sugar-laden fruit juices, and coffee. These are all foods that are very common in our diet and are considered good choices by some of the same experts who think fats are the problem. However, all of the above-named foods are known to rapidly increase the release of insulin, which starts the roller-coaster ride for our blood sugar. I am not saying that all those foods are bad, I am saying that because they trigger the release of insulin, they are going to cause your body to store fat.

The Effects of Glucagon

The second hormone we need to pay attention to when it comes to losing weight and balancing our blood sugar is glucagon. We can't control our bodies by simply talking to them and telling them to burn fats, proteins, or carbohydrates. We can't tell our bodies to burn only stored fat and leave the muscle alone. That would be just like the Tiger Woods commercial where he tells the ball to fly 350 yards with a slight fade and land softly on the green. It just doesn't happen that way, or at least not for me. We can control whether our bodies burn or store fat, but we do that by the choices we make in our diets.

There is always a triggering mechanism involved. Insulin is triggered in direct response to the amount of carbohydrates consumed. Insulin does not trigger the body to burn calories from stored body fat, it triggers the body to store fat. It also inhibits the release of glucagon, which is known to burn fat. This is why it is important to recognize which foods will work with you and which foods will be working against you in your dieting efforts.

Glucagon is a catabolic hormone. Its production is inhibited by the production of insulin. If you have a large amount of insulin circulating in the bloodstream, due to a high carbohydrate meal, your body will not be able to produce glucagon. Insulin and glucagon are at opposite ends of a teeter-totter; when one is up the other is down; and vice-versa. Therefore, if you want to be burning calories from fats it's important to trigger your body to release glucagon, which occurs by reducing your carbohydrates and increasing the consumption of proteins in your diet. I didn't say no carbohydrates; I said, reduce the number of carbohydrates. Instead of eating 70% of your calories from carbohydrates, maybe only 40–50% of your calories should come from carbohydrates. When you begin to increase the percentage of protein in your diet to 20–30%, your body will release more glucagon. Glucagon is a catabolic hormone that burns fats.

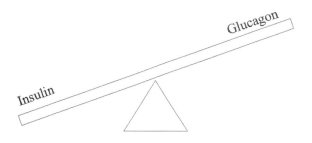

**A low-carbohydrate meal with more protein and fat
causes glucagon to increase.**

After a meal high in carbohydrates your insulin levels will skyrocket up; three to four hours pass and that insulin spike is now roller coasting down, and that's when a lot of our problems begin. Insulin is going to work to bring your blood sugar down. Unfortunately, when your blood sugar skyrockets up very fast it will usually fall just as quickly. We know that when our blood sugar is low or falling, we suffer from *food cravings, fatigue, irritability, mood swings, inability to concentrate, muscle weakness,* and the list goes on. What we need to do to promote both better health and consistent weight loss is keep our blood sugar from rising and falling so rapidly. We do this by choosing foods that have a more balanced release of both insulin and glucagon.

There are some dieting plans that say no carbohydrates, in order to release more glucagon so we can burn more fats. Well, on paper that sounds great, but in actuality we need some carbohydrates for energy and proper physiological function. Many symptoms like food cravings, irritability, light-headedness, moodiness, nervousness, and inability to think or concentrate are because the brain's only source of energy comes from the breakdown of carbohydrates (glucose). Thus, when the blood sugar is abnormally low, the brain's fuel source is also low, which causes us to function poorly. That's why it's vital to maintain a level blood sugar count.

Adrenals and Blood Sugar

We always hear how we should eat every 2–3 hours to help keep our blood sugar level. However, I think the good Lord made our bodies to be able to last more than a few hours without our blood sugar going low and causing all those symptoms associated with low blood sugar (cravings, fatigue, weight gain, irritability, inability to concentrate, muscle weakness, etc.).

This is where the adrenal glands come into play. As our blood sugar begins to drop, a signal is sent for the adrenal glands to release a hormone that will trigger our bodies to start breaking down fat into glucose (sugar). This process is meant to go on all the time, but the problem arises if our adrenal glands are exhausted and depleted. How can our adrenal glands keep our blood sugar stable and help us lose weight when they are constantly being over-stressed? Again, this takes us back to resting and nourishing our adrenal glands, because all the best dieting in the world can be negated if our cortisol levels are out of balance.

Glycemix Index

Now that you know that too many carbohydrates will trigger your body to release insulin, which stores fat, we need to learn which foods trigger the greatest insulin response and keep those foods to a minimum. A Glycemix Index will help us with this concern.

The Glycemix Index is a measurement of how quickly sugar is broken down and released into the bloodstream. Foods that release a high amount of sugar into the bloodstream are the ones that trigger the huge insulin response. These are the foods we want to stay away from or limit in our diets. Foods that are considered low or moderately low on the Glycemix Index allow for the release of glucagon, which helps stabilize our blood sugar, promotes healthy weight loss, and helps control fatigue, craving, irritability, concentration, and mood.

To help you understand the Glycemix Index, we will look at table sugar, or sucrose, because it is released very rapidly into our bloodstreams and causes a huge rise in our blood sugar levels. Foods made from refined white flour and refined white sugar cause a larger spike in our blood sugar level than unrefined flour and sugar. The carbohydrates (sugars) from an apple are released more slowly and cause a much smaller surge in our blood sugar compared to popcorn or rice cakes. Foods that are high in protein and fat (pecans, seeds, eggs, meat, chicken, fish) do not contain many carbohydrates and will not cause much of a spike in our blood sugar levels.

The name of the game is to select more of your foods from the chart below that are known to cause a low to moderate surge in your blood sugar level. You may be surprised to find out many of the foods you have been eating are foods that may be working against your natural hormonal response. What you will typically find is that foods that come in a box or package usually trigger a larger release of insulin than raw fruits and vegetables.

Glycemix Index Chart

Foods are rated according to how fast the carbohydrates are broken down and cause our blood sugar level to rise. To better control our blood sugar levels, it is recommended to eat foods from the Low and Medium categories and consume only on occasion the foods from the High and Very High categories.

Glycemix Ratings: L = Low, M = Medium, H = High, VH = Very High.

Low

Apples, Asparagus, Broccoli, Celery, Cherries, Cucumbers, Fructose, Grapefruit, Green Peppers, Lettuce, Onions, Peaches, Pears, Plums, Spinach, Strawberries, Tomatoes, Zucchini

Medium

Baked Beans, Cantaloupe, Grapes, Lactose, Oatmeal, Oranges, Pasta, Peaches, Pears, Pineapples, Pinto Beans, Sweet Potatoes, Watermelons, Yams

High

Bagels, Bananas, Bread, Cereals (Whole Grains), Carrots, Corn/Corn Chips, Muffins, Granola, Porridge, White Potatoes, Pretzels, Raisins, Rice, Sucrose, Tortillas/Tortilla Chips

Very High

Cereals (Processed/Refined), Glucose, Honey, Maltose, Plain Crackers, Popcorn, Rice Cakes, White Bread

With a basic knowledge and better understanding of how the body functions, we can now look at why the American diet has failed and why the rate of heart disease, stroke, diabetes, and obesity is on the rise. Most Americans are told to eat more carbohydrates and less fat in their diet. People are choosing to eat low fat or no fat and are replacing those calories with additional carbohydrates. This high ratio of carbohydrates to fats and proteins leads to an increased surge of insulin, which stores fat. The body can only use so many carbohydrates at one time. Additional carbohydrates are converted to fat. The large amount of sugar in our bloodstreams will trigger the body to release huge amounts of insulin. The constant huge amounts of insulin (hyperinsulinema) being released into our bloodstreams inhibits the release of glucagon. No glucagon, no fat burning! No fat burning means no long-term success on a weight loss program.

Stress, Blood Sugar, and Weight Loss

Balancing our blood sugar is vital to promote healthy weight loss. It is extremely important if you are also suffering from Stage Two or Three of functional adrenal exhaustion. If you feel that you have overtaxed your adrenal glands, it is important to eliminate or reduce the use of refined sugars from your diet. A diet high in refined carbohydrates will only exaggerate the stress on your adrenal glands. Large fluctuations in your blood sugar will only cause your adrenal glands to work harder.

The stress hormone, cortisol, has a profound effect on our blood sugar, because it combats the effectiveness of insulin. This leads to an even greater production of insulin that eventually leads to insulin resistance and/or increasing our susceptibility to diabetes. Insulin resistance is when the cells of your body are unable to recognize the insulin molecules. This is typically a result of a long history of a diet high in refined carbohydrates. The huge amount of insulin in our blood sugar causes the cells to become more resistant to insulin, which in turn leads to further production of insulin. It is that constant surge of insulin that is damaging to our health, and it is a diet loaded with refined carbohydrates that continues that cycle.

FYI: Many people who suffer from Type II adult onset diabetes are taking medications not because their pancreas isn't making enough insulin, but rather their pancreas cannot keep on making the huge amounts of insulin required by a diet high in refined carbohydrates. This is why diet and exercise can control diabetes. If you're not causing your blood sugar to surge very high, your body won't have to produce so much insulin. Secondly, when you exercise (walking is a great exercise), you make the cells of your body more receptive to insulin, which helps keep your blood sugar from going too high.

Summary

- 60% of the benefits from exercise come from our diet.
- Fats are not the main problem that causes weight gain.
- Controlling blood sugar levels helps your weight loss efforts.
- The types of foods we eat will determine our blood sugar level.
- Insulin is produced in response to carbohydrates in the diet.
- Insulin promotes the storage of fats.
- Glucagon promotes the breakdown of fats.
- Insulin inhibits the release of glucagon.
- Choose foods from the Glycemix Index that are considered low to moderate with regard to their release of insulin.

Action Steps

- Evaluate which hormones you trigger when you eat.
- Choose foods that promote blood sugar stability.
- Reduce or eliminate refined carbohydrates from your diet.

Chapter Six

The Five and Two Plan

If you take five steps forward and take two steps back, how much progress have you made? Obviously, you've taken three steps forward overall. Sure, you would be closer to your goal if you had not taken two steps back, but it would have been worse if you had taken five steps back and made no progress at all.

I would like to use that same philosophy and apply it to a weekly dieting plan. Five days treat your body like a temple and two days treat it like an amusement park. What I mean is, for five days follow a healthy, balanced, nutritious diet that will regulate your blood sugar and promote healthy weight loss. Then, if you need to take a break and reward yourself for five days of good eating, you can go ahead and eat less healthy on two days. I call it the Five and Two Plan. Most people find it easier to eat healthy during the week, and reward themselves with desserts and other junk foods that are not meant to promote good health during the weekend.

The goal is to have more good days of dieting than bad days. When you start doing that, you will start making some progress with your weight loss efforts. If we diet well for five days and do poorly for two days, at least we had more good days of dieting than bad. We take more steps in the right direction with our diets by choosing to have more good days of dieting than bad. Of course it would be better to have seven days of healthy eating for better health and well-being, but for some of us mental anguish and feelings of deprivation and boredom take over our thinking. So, let yourself go and enjoy the times that you get to go to the "amusement park" of dieting.

Another way to look at this dieting approach on a daily basis is to consider how well you would do if you had a great, nutritious breakfast, a terrible lunch, and a fairly poor dinner. When you add that all up, it sounds like you took one step forward and two steps back. In other words, you made no progress in your desire to lose weight and become healthier. The object of the game is to eat more healthy meals and take steps forward in your diet program. When you are able to do this consistently, you will do a better job of reaching your weight loss goals.

I've also learned that when people do a good job of dieting for five days, they oftentimes look forward to rewarding themselves with something sinfully delicious on those two other days. The goal is to treat your body like a temple and diet well for five days, then you feel justified for earning your reward with an amusement park day. You can't or you shouldn't go to the amusement (sweets, cookies, candies, desserts, junk food, etc. . . .) park every day; you need to earn that right. Therefore, treat your body right for five days and earn the trips to the amusement park.

For centuries people have lived healthy lives without the need of counting calories or weighing out their portions. I don't believe in making people do more for themselves than I would do for myself. Therefore, if you follow the simple Five and Two Plan I've described and follow the ten steps I've outlined below in your everyday life, you will begin to lose weight and get healthier.

Ten Steps for Healthy Eating

1. **Regulate your blood sugar by controlling insulin and glucagon.**
2. **Reduce or eliminate refined white flour and sugars from your diet.**
3. **Eat a fiber-rich diet.**
4. **Avoid partially hydrogenated fats, artificial sweeteners, preservatives, and artificially colored foods.**
5. **Raw nuts, seeds, and fruits are excellent snack foods.**
6. **Drink only a few ounces of water with your meal.**

7. Eat organic foods as much as possible.
8. Combine your foods appropriately.
9. Don't ruin a healthy, nutritious meal with an unhealthy dessert.
10. Relax and enjoy your meal.

Step One—Regulate your blood sugar by controlling insulin and glucagon.
- Eat good protein and fats with each meal.
- Proteins stimulate the release of glucagon.
- Dietary fats slow the release of insulin into your bloodstream.
- Some protein-rich foods are eggs, chicken, seafood, beef, pork, lamb, and wild game.
- Glucagon promotes the breakdown of fats.
- The monounsaturated fats (omega-3 and omega-6) are good fats to eat.
- Good fats are found in coldwater fish (salmon, mackerel, halibut, cod, sardines), nuts and seeds, and various oils (olive, flax, canola, sesame, safflower, evening primrose, and cod liver oil).

Step Two—Reduce or eliminate refined white flour and white sugar.
- Foods that are made with processed flours and sugars trigger a larger release of insulin and throw your blood sugar further out of balance.
- Most prepackaged food is highly refined. Stay away from foods that come in a box or wrapped in plastic.
- Foods that are made with highly refined white flour and sugar should be replaced with 100% whole grain, unrefined foods.

Step Three—Eat a diet rich in fiber.
- Constipation is the unspoken common problem of today that causes internal pollution of your body.
- Eat a raw salad a day.
- Eat 5–7 servings of fruits, vegetables, and whole grains per day.
- Use a natural fiber supplement that doesn't have added sugars or artificial sweeteners.

Step Four—Avoid partially hydrogenated fats, artificial sweeteners and preservatives.
- Partially hydrogenated fats are found in many baked and prepackaged food.
- They have been chemically altered from their natural state and are more difficult for the body to process.
- Margarine is a partially hydrogenated fat. Butter is better.
- Artificial sweeteners have not shown any proof that they contribute to weight loss, and many people show sensitivity to these artificial sweeteners.
- Artificial preservatives, colors, dyes, and flavoring are all chemicals that we are ingesting and which contribute to chemical stress.

Step Five—Nuts, seeds, and fruits make excellent snacks.
- Almonds, pecans, walnuts, macadamias, cashews, sunflower seeds, flax seeds, etc. . . . are a great source of omega-3 and -6 fatty acids.
- Nuts and seeds can easily be added to cereal, oatmeal, and yogurt to help slow down the release of insulin from a meal loaded with carbohydrates.
- Fruits are better to eat by themselves.
- Many people are sensitive to peanuts; stay away from peanuts if you suspect candida or fungal yeast overgrowth.

Step Six—Drink only a few ounces (2–6 ounces) of water with your meal.
- The body produces enzymes to digest and break down food.
- When we ingest large amounts of fluids with our meals (water, tea, soda, coffee, or juices), we dilute the concentration and effectiveness of these enzymes.
- Bloating, gas, heartburn, indigestion, or reflux could be caused by excessive fluid consumption.
- Drink 8–10 glasses of water a day; just don't drink them with your meals.

Step Seven—Eat as much organic and unrefined food as possible.
- Since the Garden of Eden we have eaten organic food.
- Foods loaded with antibiotics, insecticides, pesticides, and other harsh chemicals are taxing to the body.

- Organic foods have a higher percentage of vitamins and minerals than non-organic foods.

Step Eight—Combine your foods properly.
- Certain foods combine better than other foods.
- Proteins do not combine well with starchy carbohydrates (potatoes, corn, rice, beans, breads). This does not mean they cannot be eaten together, only that it is more difficult to digest them.
- Proteins combine well with fibrous vegetables (broccoli, spinach, asparagus, squash, zucchini, and other green, leafy vegetables).
- Eat fruits by themselves.
- Proper food combining can eliminate and reduce irritable bowel, leaky gut, indigestion, bloating, gas, and heartburn.
- No other animal on earth eats as humans do. We like to have five or six different foods on our plate; yet in nature, animals will stop and eat a whole carcass, a whole bunch of leaves, or a stalk of bananas at one time. This makes digestion much easier.

Step Nine—Don't ruin a healthy, nutritious meal with a bad dessert.
- You are what your body absorbs!
- Don't assume that if you ate it your body absorbed it.
- Other unspoken common complaints are bloating, gas, indigestion, and heartburn.
- The absorption of a nutritious, healthy meal can be hampered by food sensitivities and/or the addition of a dessert that is loaded with refined sugars, chemicals, sweeteners, flavors, and dyes.
- If you want to have a dessert, wait at least an hour and eat it by itself or splurge on your amusement park day.
- Common food sensitivities are dairy, wheat, corn, soy, coffee, and tea.

Step Ten—Relax and enjoy your meal.
- Eating on the run, in a hurry, or standing up hinders absorption and can inhibit the production of digestive enzymes, which leads to bloating, gas, indigestion, and heartburn.
- Take the time to enjoy your meal and properly digest your food.

Balancing Carbohydrates, Proteins, and Fats

The key to healthy dieting begins with balancing and regulating your blood sugar. A meal high in carbohydrates will trigger the release of insulin. Stay away from foods that are rated "high" and "very high" on the Glycemix Index. When fewer carbohydrates and more proteins and fats are eaten, the hormone glucagon is released, which promotes the breakdown of fats. Glucagon works at breaking down fats, while insulin works to store fats.

Breakfast—It is called breakfast because when you think about it you are actually "breaking" a mini "fast." Many people choose to skip, scrimp, or choose the wrong foods to start their day. Those who skip breakfast completely are making the biggest mistake. Breakfast or lunch should be your largest meal of the day. If most people have their last meal of the day no later than eight or nine in the evening and then skip breakfast and don't eat until mid-morning, they may go 12–14 hours without putting any type of nourishment in their bodies. Our blood sugar is typically lowest in the morning, since we haven't eaten anything for approximately 10 to 12 hours. That's a half-day fast! Therefore, we need to "break" that mini fast in the morning with a meal that will nourish our bodies with enough calories and energy to make our day productive and keep our blood sugar in balance.

Patient Story

Alex was a young, healthy 32-year-old who complained of fatigue, irritability, and anxiety. He was very athletic and followed a very clean diet. He didn't eat much junk food and ate lots of good proteins, fats, and carbohydrates. In the mornings he followed a very intense and demanding workout six days a week. He typically didn't eat after 8 P.M.; he wouldn't eat anything before his workout, and he wouldn't complete his workout until 8 A.M. He would have a cup of coffee on his way to work and would not eat until mid-morning, if at all.

Since he waited to eat his first meal of the day at mid-morning his blood sugar was completely depleted, due to the fact that he hadn't eaten since 8 P.M. the night before. Plus, he further compounded that problem with an intense workout that further depleted his blood sugar.

After reviewing this regimen, I suggested he eat some fruit in the morning and wait at least 20 minutes before starting his morning workout. I also advised him to start having breakfast after his workout in order to replenish his blood sugar and nourish his body. His lack of energy, irritability, and anxiety were associated with the low blood sugar caused by his workout and his dietary choices. His complaints lessened when he started to maintain his blood sugar levels.

If you complain of low blood sugar, food cravings, lack of energy, irritability, and moodiness if meals are missed or delayed, it is extremely important to get a good start to your day, and not let your blood sugar roller coaster up and down by missing breakfast or eating a meal that is loaded with carbohydrates. The everyday cup of coffee and/or bagel for breakfast sends your blood sugar sky high and starts that roller-coaster ride the rest of the day with your blood sugar.

Carbohydrates will also trigger the release of various brain messengers that have a very sedative, calming, and relaxing effect on the brain. A meal with more protein triggers brain messengers that have a stimulatory and excitatory effect on the brain. This is important particularly if you have a big presentation or test to take, because you need to be thinking as clearly as possible. The last thing you want to do is trigger brain messengers that are going to make your thinking sedate, calm, and slow. Therefore, eat a meal that contains more protein and fewer carbohydrates in order to promote a more alert, excited response.

Meal Suggestions

Breakfast—Eggs are a great choice and can be made so many ways.
- Poached, soft-boiled, hard-boiled, scrambled, fried, or omelets.
- Omelets are my preferred choice, with plenty of vegetables (onions, garlic, cilantro, jalapeños, or any veggie you prefer).
- Quiche is another great choice, made with plenty of vegetables.
- Whole grain (100%) cereals or oatmeal is another great breakfast choice.
- I recommend eating these carbohydrate-rich foods with a handful of nuts, such as almonds, pecans, walnuts, macadamias, pine, or any other kind of nut.
- The fats found in nuts and seeds slow down the release of sugar into our bloodstreams. Therefore, whenever eating a food that is considered high or very high on the Glycemix Index, add a small handful of nuts to slow down the release of sugar. This keeps the insulin from surging so high and helps keep our blood sugar from getting out of balance.

Lunch—To avoid that mid-afternoon drop in energy, stay away from a meal loaded with carbohydrates. A combination of protein (fish, chicken, beef, egg, tuna, lamb, or pork) and green, leafy vegetables makes an excellent meal.

- Grilled chicken salad, taco salad (avoid the shell), shrimp salad, a salad with a couple of eggs.
- Beef, fish, chicken, tuna with a large salad.
- Beef, fish, chicken, tuna with two to three servings of vegetables (broccoli, spinach, squash, and other green, leafy vegetables).
- Homemade chili, made with little or no beans.
- Fajitas (beef or chicken), enchiladas and tacos can be eaten, but limit the intake of beans and rice and avoid fried tortilla chips.
- Don't be afraid of avocados! We are not a nation of overweight people because we eat too many avocados.
- Beef stew; try to minimize the starchy carbohydrates (potatoes, corn, and carrots) and add some other vegetables.
- Chinese food is fine, but limit the noodles and rice and eat plenty of vegetables.
- With Italian food, include protein and limit the pasta.

Dinner—Dinner should be the smallest of your three meals. Unfortunately, it is typically the largest meal for most people. Dinner is usually an extension of lunch. If you want to add more carbohydrates to your meal, let it be at dinner. Remember, carbohydrates promote calmness, sedation, and relaxation in your body, which is what is needed when we begin to unwind and relax, when we finish a long day and prepare for bedtime.

Snacks—Should be anything healthy (nuts, seeds, and fruits are great choices).

Summary

- Follow the Five and Two Plan.
- Treat your body like a temple for five days and treat it like an amusement park for two days.
- Eat more good meals than bad meals in a week.
- The more good meals you have in a week compared to bad meals will show how well you are doing with your diet.
- Take more steps forward in the right direction with your diet.

Action Steps

- Learn the Ten Steps for Healthy Dieting and follow them!

Chapter Seven

Exercise and Fitness

A question often asked is: Do you need to exercise in order to lose weight and keep it off? No, you don't have to exercise to lose weight, but if you want to complement your dieting efforts it will definitely help speed up the process. A second question asked is: Will my body firm up and tone up as I start to lose weight? No, you will have to do some type of exercise if you want to add shape and tone to your body.

The first point I need to make about an exercise program is: I am not trying to make anybody an athlete! An exercise program is anything as simple as walking, stretching, or yoga. The more serious athlete may include jogging, cycling, swimming, aerobic dance, or weight training. My goal is to incorporate physical activity into your lifestyle that will lead to better health and fitness. Are you an athlete or someone who already incorporates some sort of training into your schedule but are not receiving the results you think you should? This section will help educate you on what happens to the body when you exercise and what type of exercises may be beneficial to get the desired look while at the same time becoming healthier.

As you recall, good fitness and good health are two different things. The focus is to design an exercise program that promotes good fitness as well as good health. Since the main point of this book is how our hormones trigger our bodies to either burn or store fat, we will discuss which types of physical exercise trigger the body to burn calories from fat and which trigger the body to burn calories from proteins and carbohydrates.

Manufacturing Energy

All along we've been talking about the importance of burning calories from fats as opposed to proteins and carbohydrates to succeed in any weight loss program. To produce energy, we must first break down fats, proteins and carbohydrates into a useable form of energy. The breakdown of one gram of fat burns nine calories while the breakdown of one gram of protein or carbohydrate burns only four calories. Fat burns roughly two and a half times more calories than protein or carbohydrate. It's important to understand that the breakdown of carbohydrates into energy is quicker than protein or fats, but the supply is limited. Additional biochemical steps are needed to break down proteins and fats. All three will eventually be broken down into adenosine triphosphate (ATP), which is the actual currency used for the production of energy.

To better understand how the body chooses to burn calories, I'm going to use a different analogy than the fireplace story. So, imagine the way your body breaks down fat, proteins and carbohydrates to produce energy (ATP), as different types of financial assets. Think of carbohydrates as money in your checking account; it's easily accessible and can quickly be used as cash. It's limited in supply because you should have more stashed away in a long-term savings or retirement account, which is what fats can be thought of as. If you need to tap into your retirement account to get cash you can, but it's not as easily accessible as your checking account.

The point is that carbohydrates are easily converted into cash (energy), while the money in your savings accounts (fats) is not as easily converted into cash. A good financial planner will tell you that you should have more money socked away in a retirement account than in a simple checking account. The body is quite similar; we have more potential energy from the fat on our bodies than from the available carbohydrates because their supply is limited. Now we come to where the similarities of our financial model differ, because we don't ever want to use money that has been saved in our retirement account, but we do want to use the fat stored away on our bodies for energy.

Continuing with our financial analogy, there is an exchange rate that comes into play when we produce energy (ATP). This is where exercise and the intensity level you train at can have an impact on the production of energy (ATP). One molecule of glucose (sugar) is broken down and converted into either two ATPs or 36 ATPs. The deciding factor for that conversion rate is dependent on the availability of oxygen. It's definitely smarter to exchange one glucose molecule for 36 ATPs than it is for only two ATPs. Therefore, the buying power of energy is greater when oxygen is available.

If the exercise intensity level is low to moderate and oxygen is available, the body will use "aerobic metabolism" to produce energy. This allows for the conversion of 36 units of energy. However, if the intensity level is high enough that it reduces the availability of oxygen, the body will produce energy by way of "anaerobic metabolism." This method is less efficient and only produces two units of energy.

I hope I haven't lost you, but the point to remember is that oxygen is needed if we want to burn calories from fats when we exercise. This is why it is important to examine the intensity level of your workout. Depending on the level, the intensity of your workout determines if there is oxygen available or not. If your intensity level is too hard when you work out, you may not have enough oxygen available to burn calories from fat.

A drawback that comes from burning calories from carbohydrates without oxygen is a byproduct called lactic acid. Think of lactic acid as the "interest rate" that needs to be paid back. If there is a high accumulation of lactic acid, fatigue sets in. A high interest rate will wear anybody down. This is why it is important to examine the intensity level, because if you're only producing two units of energy instead of 36 units, you may run out of energy very quickly. However, if the intensity level is low to moderate, which allows for the availability of oxygen, you produce 36 units of energy. There is no high interest to be paid, therefore less fatigue is experienced, but most importantly we can burn calories from stored body fat.

Aerobic and Anaerobic Metabolism

The workouts you do can be classified as either aerobic or anaerobic exercises. The intensity level you train at will trigger your body to either use aerobic or anaerobic metabolism.

The term "aerobic exercise" is a fairly common term, which most people are familiar with. Most people think of aerobic exercise as any physical activity such as walking, running, cycling, stair-climbing, aerobic dance, or swimming for 10, 20, 30 minutes or more, at a low to moderate intensity level.

Anaerobic exercise, on the other hand, is an activity like weight lifting, sprinting, speed skating, or any type of physical activity that can be done for only a very short period of time and at a much higher level of intensity. This type of activity cannot be sustained for long periods of time.

Aerobic and anaerobic metabolism is the process the body uses to produce energy. Aerobic literally means with oxygen, while anaerobic means without oxygen. If oxygen is available because your aerobic exercise was done at low to moderate intensity, "aerobic metabolism" will trigger the body to burn calories from fats. However, if oxygen is unavailable because of high intensity training, "anaerobic metabolism" is used and the body will burn calories from the breakdown of carbohydrates and proteins for energy.

One of the main reasons for our inability to firm and tone our bodies through exercising is that many of us are performing aerobic activities at too high an intensity level, which triggers "anaerobic metabolism." In other words, we are doing aerobic activities such as walking, jogging, cycling, stair-climbing, dancing, and swimming at a higher intensity level than our bodies are conditioned for. Thus, our bodies are depending on "anaerobic metabolism" for the production of energy instead of "aerobic metabolism." This causes our bodies to burn calories from carbohydrates and proteins, and not fat. In which case people are sometimes misled into thinking that because they are burning calories, they are burning calories from stored body fat. They may think they are losing weight, but they are actually burning lean muscle tissue (protein), not fat. If you have a hard time adding shape and tone to your body, it could be because you're burning muscle and not fat for energy when you work out.

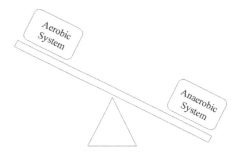

Low intensity exercise causes aerobic metabolism to dominate.

Both aerobic and anaerobic metabolism function simultaneously throughout the day; they are literally inversely related, meaning when one system is up, the other is down, and vice-versa. The key point to remember is that as the intensity of your aerobic workout increases, your availability of oxygen decreases. Let me explain. As you go from walking to jogging to running, you will become more and more out of breath and start breathing more and more heavily. The reason you are breathing heavier is because you are trying to get more oxygen into your lungs to carry to your muscles.

If you are sitting around reading, you're probably producing most of your energy through aerobic metabolism, but if you are running from that saber-toothed tiger, your body will be predominantly running off of anaerobic metabolism. If you were to begin to walk down the street, your body would begin to use a little more of its anaerobic metabolism and a bit less of its aerobic metabolism, and you would notice that your breathing had increased. If you start jogging down the street, your body will use even less of your aerobic metabolism and more of your anaerobic metabolism and your breathing will become even more intense. Now, if you start to run, your body will probably use nothing but anaerobic metabolism and your breathing will become very rapid and intense. What we will talk about later is determining the aerobic threshold or plateau (intensity level which is measured by our heart rate) we can exercise at that allows us to continually use aerobic metabolism.

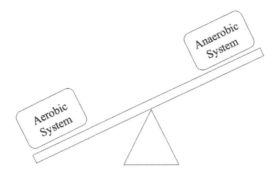

High intensity exercise causes anaerobic metabolism to dominate.

A major difference in these two systems is that aerobic metabolism takes a little longer to produce energy than anaerobic metabolism. Just as in the analogy about money, anaerobic metabolism quickly converts carbohydrates (checking account) into readily available currency (ATP), whereas aerobic metabolism utilizes fats (long-term retirement savings account), and takes longer to convert into energy (ATP).

Now let's talk about the differences between aerobic and anaerobic exercise. Aerobic exercise typically means with oxygen, whereas anaerobic exercise is without oxygen. Aerobic exercise is low to moderate intensity for a prolonged period of time, while anaerobic exercise is typically done at high intensity over a short period of time. If you're training aerobically, you're able to supply your body (muscles) with as much oxygen as the body is demanding. However, when you train anaerobically your muscles are demanding more oxygen than you're able to supply.

It's all a matter of supply and demand. If you're training at low to moderate intensity, your body is not demanding a huge supply of oxygen. Therefore, your body can easily supply enough oxygen, which enables your body to burn calories from fats. However, as you increase the intensity of your aerobic workout, your muscles begin to demand more oxygen. As the intensity increases further, you will reach a point where you can't supply enough oxygen to your muscles as is needed. When that happens you go into what is referred to as "oxygen debt." When you're in oxygen debt, your muscles are dependent on anaerobic metabolism for energy. When there is no oxygen available due to intense training, you're not going to be burning calories from stored body fats. It's the intensity of your aerobic training that will determine if your body is burning calories from fats or from carbohydrates and proteins. We will discuss more about finding the proper training intensity to ensure our aerobic system is being utilized properly.

An important piece of the puzzle regarding exercise and weight loss is the availability of oxygen. Too often people do aerobic exercise at so high an intensity level for their level of conditioning that they trigger anaerobic metabolism because they don't have any oxygen available. If there is no oxygen available, your body can only break down carbohydrates and proteins. If there is no oxygen available there is no fat breakdown! This can explain why so many people are not losing weight and firming up from all the calories they're burning when they exercise. It doesn't really matter how many calories you're burning, if you're only burning calories from carbohydrates and protein. Don't forget, we don't want to break down proteins for energy; we're exercising to add lean muscle tissue.

The last difference between the two is: aerobic exercise is easy to perform as well as stress reducing; while anaerobic exercise is more taxing and stress producing. Recall that physical stress is another component that can exhaust the adrenal glands. It's possible your training routine may be contributing to your adrenal exhaustion, which leads to the inability to burn fat and lose weight.

How do you feel when you finish your aerobic workout? Do you feel good and refreshed or are you tired and fatigued? A good rule of thumb to use after completing your aerobic workout (walking, jogging, stair-steps, cycling, aerobic dance, etc.), is to ask yourself if you can do the exact same workout, all over again, at that moment. If you can say yes, you probably trained aerobically. If you feel exhausted and tired after your aerobic activity, you may be training at too high an intensity level, which is making your body burn up all the available carbohydrates. Anaerobic metabolism produces a lot of lactic acid, which makes you feel fatigued and exhausted. The hardest thing to make someone understand is that unless you are training for some competition, you don't need to be killing yourself when you do your aerobic workout.

Training Intensity

The goal of aerobic training should be to keep your intensity level at such a rate that it allows aerobic metabolism. When we do that we expand our aerobic capacity and better utilize fats for energy. This is a very important function of overall cardiovascular health.

FYI: If you are following a low- or no-carbohydrate diet and your exercise intensity is too high, you're forced to use anaerobic metabolism. There is a good chance you are burning lean muscle tissue when you exercise. This is because there is no oxygen available, which doesn't allow fat to be burned. Second, whatever carbohydrates that were available may be quickly used up; therefore, you have no more carbohydrates to burn. When this happens, the body only has one option—it can't burn fat or carbohydrates—so it burns proteins (lean muscle tissue). This is the last thing we want to do when we exercise.

Summary

Aerobic exercise
- Stress reducing
- Can be performed for long periods of time
- Supplies oxygen
- Promotes the breakdown of fats for energy.

Anaerobic exercise
- Stress producing
- Can only be done for short periods of time
- Is performed without oxygen
- Breaks down carbohydrates and proteins for energy
- Produces lactic acid and fatigue.

Aerobic metabolism
- Requires oxygen
- Burns fat for energy
- Produces 36 units of energy.

Anaerobic metabolism
- Does not require oxygen
- Burns carbohydrates and proteins
- Produces 2 units of energy.

Action Steps

- Adjust your aerobic training intensity to meet your health goals.

Chapter Eight

Target Fat-Burning Zone

We have all heard of the proverbial fat-burning zone. But what is it? Is it different for each person? Are you training in your fat-burning zone? Are you doing your aerobic training at too high an intensity level? Could you be over-training?

The intensity level of your workout is measured by your heart rate. The faster your heart beats, the more intense the workout. As you walk, run, cycle, swim, or dance faster, your heart rate increases. When you walk, run, cycle, swim, or dance slower, your heart rate decreases. Therefore, the more intense the workout, the faster your heart beats.

The name of the game is to train aerobically by keeping the intensity of your workout low to moderate. When we do that we trigger aerobic metabolism and burn fat for energy. The problem is that most people do their aerobic training at too high an intensity level, which triggers anaerobic metabolism. We tend to think that we are in better shape aerobically than we actually are. This causes us to train at a higher intensity level than we should. If your aerobic workout is being fueled by anaerobic metabolism, you will be triggering the breakdown of carbohydrates and proteins (muscle) for energy, not fats! If you're not getting the results you want from your training regimen, it's time to start measuring your intensity level to determine if you are utilizing aerobic metabolism. The results may surprise you.

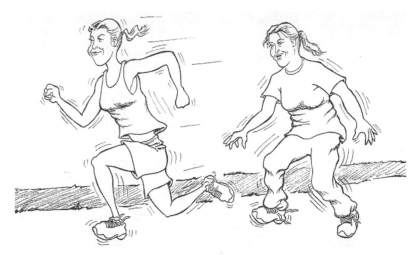

Two people running at the same speed does not mean they are exercising at the same intensity.

Different Intensity Levels

We are told the fat-burning zone is a range or percentage of our maximum heart rate. This is true! However, each person's fat-burning zone is different, depending on each person's level of conditioning. The charts say a 40-year-old person will be aerobic if they train between 55–85% of their maximum heart rate. That doesn't mean that one 40-year-old who has been a couch potato can train at the same target heart rate as another 40-year-old who has been an avid runner for years and receive the same benefits. Their target fat-burning zones could be at different levels.

If they both train at 75% of their maximum heart rate, the first guy will probably be training at too high an intensity level and be dependent on anaerobic metabolism, which will not give him the fat-burning benefits he is after. He will be adding more physical stress to his body, which leads to fatigue caused by lactic acid, because his fat-burning zone is probably only at 70% of his maximum heart rate. On the other hand, the one who has been training for years can probably exercise at 75% of his maximum heart rate and still be in his fat-burning zone. He's burning calories from fats, he's not feeling fatigued after his workout, and he is reducing stress.

In order to determine what your target fat-burning zone is, it would be good to get an idea what your maximum heart rate is. This is determined by subtracting your age from 220. For example a 40-year-old individual has a maximum heart rate of 180 (220 minus 40 equals 180) beats per minute.

Intensity level and aerobic metabolism are inversely related, just as aerobic and anaerobic metabolism are inversely related. When one is up, the other is down, and vice-versa. When the intensity of our workout increases, our aerobic metabolism decreases.

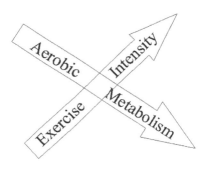

As exercise intensity increases, aerobic metabolism decreases.

Let's take, for example, a 40-year-old person with a resting heart rate of 65 beats per minute (bpm). His resting heart rate is 36% (65 divided by 180 equals 36%) of his maximum heart rate. As he begins to walk, his heart rate increases to 100 bpm, which is 56% (100 divided by 180 equals 56%) of his maximum heart rate. Since his intensity level has increased (from sitting to walking), he is depending a little more on his anaerobic metabolism and a little less on his aerobic metabolism, as compared to when he was at rest. When he begins to jog, his heart rate increases to 140 bpm, which is 77% (140 divided by 180 equals 77%) of his maximum heart rate. He's now using a great percentage of anaerobic metabolism and a smaller percentage of aerobic metabolism, all because there is less oxygen available due to the increase of the intensity of the exercise. If he begins to run faster, his heart rate increases to 160 bpm, which is 89% (160 divided by 180 equals 89%) of the maximum intensity his heart can beat. When he is training at this

101

intensity level, he is probably getting 100% of his energy from anaerobic metabolism and nothing from aerobic metabolism.

The important thing to realize is that the intensity level determines which of the two systems is predominantly used. As the intensity level, measured by your heart rate, increases, your anaerobic metabolism will be responsible for a greater percentage of energy than your aerobic metabolism. The more intense a workout, the greater percentage of calories is burned from carbohydrates than from fats. Lower intensity workouts allow for more fat to be burned for calories than carbohydrates. This is one of the reasons why walking is such a great activity for promoting better health and fitness. Of course, you will burn more calories when you run, cycle, swim or dance harder, but were all those calories you burned coming from the breakdown of fats or carbohydrates?

Aerobic Threshold

Every person has what is called a maxVO2 or aerobic threshold, which is the maximum amount of intensity someone can train at and still have oxygen in his or her tissues. We measure intensity levels with our heart rates and as our heart rates increase, our availability of oxygen decreases. Our aerobic threshold is that point where these two lines intersect. Once your intensity level takes you over this aerobic threshold, your body burns calories almost exclusively from carbohydrates through anaerobic metabolism. As long as you train below this aerobic threshold, oxygen is present and your aerobic metabolism will function to burn calories from fats. *The goal should be to train no higher than your aerobic threshold.*

Confusion arises because each person's aerobic threshold is different. The thought that you can train anywhere between 55–85% of your maximum heart rate and be aerobic is true, but we are all different and each person will have a different aerobic threshold based on our aerobic fitness. We need to find out where that level of intensity (aerobic threshold) is and train within those guidelines. If you're training above your aerobic threshold, you're probably not triggering your body to burn calories from fat, due to the lack of oxygen.

If there is no oxygen readily available while you work out, the body's ability to burn calories from fat ceases and the body looks for another source of fuel to burn. If all the carbohydrates are used up, and there is still no oxygen available, the body begins to burn calories from the breakdown of protein (lean muscle tissue). This should explain why many of us are doing hours upon hours of both aerobic and anaerobic (weight training) exercise and not seeing our bodies tone up. You could be doing your aerobic training at too high an intensity level that's causing the breakdown of only carbohydrates and protein, which can easily lead to over-training.

A common mistake that happens when people work out at too high an intensity level or over-train is they oftentimes break down lean muscle tissue instead of fat. This mistake can be quite deceiving because it is easy to assume that any weight loss that occurs is the result of fat loss. This may not be the case. Although many people will be happy to see themselves lighter the next time they weigh themselves, they could actually be breaking down lean muscle tissue, which is heavier than fat, and creating a false sense of success in their weight loss efforts.

We discussed earlier how eating a diet that is too restrictive in carbohydrates can be damaging and can trigger the wrong hormonal responses. People who are following a low-carbohydrate diet and are exercising at too high an intensity level may be unknowingly burning calories from lean muscle tissue due to their training regimens. If you recall, carbohydrates are in limited supply in the body. If you are restricting the consumption of carbohydrates and are exercising at an intensity level that depletes all your available carbohydrates, your body will be forced to burn lean muscle tissue for energy. It's like a multiple-choice question. If I have a limited amount of carbohydrates and I train anaerobically, what is my body going to burn for energy? Well, since it's anaerobic metabolism there is no fat burning. I've used up all my carbohydrates, so the answer is my body will burn lean muscle tissue for energy. Unfortunately, that's not what we want to be doing when we

Patient Story

Thomas had been following a low-carbohydrate diet for almost a year and was pleased that he had lost over 50 pounds. He had been running three times a week for 30–45 minutes and weight trained for 45 minutes, three days a week. However, he had hit a plateau for the last three months and was frustrated because he couldn't understand why he wasn't able to add any shape and tone to his body.

After reviewing his diet and monitoring his aerobic workout, we increased his consumption of carbohydrates by adding a piece of fruit to his daily diet and allowed an additional carbohydrate snack on the days he weight trained. We found that he was performing his aerobic training at too high an intensity level. Instead of running for 30–45 minutes and feeling exhausted, he began to walk at a pace that kept his heart rate below his aerobic threshold. He complained about having to exercise at such a slow speed, but within two short weeks he noticed his energy increased, he didn't have that mental fog after his workouts, and he finally started seeing some muscular definition in his arms and chest.

Thomas had been training at an intensity level that was depleting the limited amount of carbohydrates in his body. Since his workouts were intense, he was causing his body to burn calories from protein (lean muscle tissue) and not fat. His aerobic workouts were now burning fats for energy and not lean muscle tissue. This made him look leaner and he once again felt like he was getting some results for all his efforts in the gym.

exercise. Just because you lost weight, don't automatically assume the weight you lost came from the breakdown of fats.

The questions we need to ask ourselves are: Are we doing our aerobic training at or below our aerobic thresholds (target fat-burning zone) to ensure the breakdown of fats? Where is our target fat-burning zone? Are we doing our aerobic exercises at too high an intensity level?

Finding Your Fat-Burning Zone

To better understand the target fat-burning zone, we need a basic understanding of how this zone is determined. As I said before, the fat-burning zone is based on a percentage of your maximum heart rate. The simple equation of subtracting your age from 220 (220 minus age equals maximum heart rate) to determine your maximum heart rate is at best an estimate. This is a general equation and is oversimplified by assuming there are no other variables that should be considered when assessing someone's maximum heart rate, such as weight, medical history, or previous training. It's simply based on the factor of age alone. For years, people have been told that if you maintain your heart rate between 55–85% of your maximum heart rate, you are performing aerobic exercise, and this will cause the body to burn calories from stored body fat.

Generally, that is a true statement. However, as we just stated, two people who are the same age yet with different aerobic fitness levels can't work out at the same speed and expect to get the same results. Every person's fat-burning zone or aerobic threshold is different and is determined by his or her current level of fitness, not their age. If you train above your aerobic threshold or fat-burning zone, you have no oxygen available, which prevents your body from burning calories from fat. Only the most well-conditioned athletes (marathoners and triathletes) can train at 85% of their maximum heart rates and still use aerobic metabolism for the production of energy. Since most people are not as well conditioned as these athletes, they should not be doing their aerobic training at 85% of maximum heart rate. You can train at 85% of your maximum heart rate, but that doesn't mean you are training aerobically and burning calories from fat.

The aerobic threshold (target fat-burning zone) for most people is about 70% of their maximum heart rate. If you've been sedentary, overweight, not working out, and are poorly conditioned, that percentage will probably be less; it could be closer to 55% or 60%, depending on your current health condition. Realize that as you consistently train aerobically you will expand your aerobic capacity and become more aerobically conditioned. This will slowly cause your aerobic threshold to rise. It doesn't occur overnight, but the more you train aerobically, the more you expand your aerobic capacity, which will slowly increase your aerobic threshold.

Going back to the assumption that we can all train between 55–85% of our maximum heart rate and be aerobic is true. Unfortunately for many of us, our egos get in the way, and we assume we can train at 80–85% of our maximum heart rate when in actuality we need to train at 70–75% of our maximum heart rate or lower to ensure that our bodies are burning calories from fats. The flip side to that ego problem is that most people don't realize they are training at that high of an intensity level. This is why I always suggest using a heart rate monitor when you do your aerobic training.

My Ego Is in the Way?

People will typically train at a high level of intensity, thinking the "no pain, no gain" philosophy is the way to obtain results. I myself used to believe the same thing and let my ego get in the way because I didn't know whether to train at 60% or 80% of my maximum heart rate. Therefore, I always chose the higher percentage!

When I first learned about training below my aerobic threshold, I had to slow my running down considerably in order to keep my heart rate within my fat-burning zone. I began to use a heart rate monitor to measure my intensity level and was amazed by how much slower I needed to be running. In fact, I hate to admit this, but I was embarrassed to run in public. I did not want anyone to see me running so slowly. My ego was used to running at a nice fast pace. I thought I was a pretty good runner, but was I in for an awakening! The whole time I was running, I was depending on anaerobic metabolism for energy. I thought as long as I was doing an aerobic activity, it must be aerobic. Was I wrong! I should have been running slower in order to promote the breakdown of fats and build my aerobic capacity.

The real eye-opener came when I stopped to think about this training method and realized I was having to run so slow to keep my heart rate below 70% of my maximum heart rate. It didn't add up! Why were my heart muscles beating so fast when my leg muscles were moving so slowly? Why did I have to jog at such a slow pace to stay within my aerobic threshold? Was I in that poor of aerobic condition? Was my aerobic capacity that low? It didn't make sense to me; I thought I was in good shape, and I could run at a pretty good pace for 20, 30, even 40 minutes. Sure, I was tired afterwards, but I thought that's what I needed to be doing in order to see any kind of results.

It wasn't until I started using a heart rate monitor that I learned I was training (intensity level) above my aerobic threshold (fat-burning zone). I had to slow my pace down to a slow jog to stay aerobic, which was very hard for me. However, this made all the difference in the world. In fact, when I ran at my normal speed I found that my heart rate was around 85% of my maximum. If you recall, only those well-conditioned athletes, marathoners, and triathletes who have properly conditioned themselves can train at up to 85% of their maximum heart rates and still trigger aerobic metabolism. Unfortunately for me, I wasn't a well-conditioned runner and was always training anaerobically, which was triggering the breakdown of carbohydrates and lean muscle tissue, not fats.

Within a few weeks of proper aerobic training, I began to notice how much leaner I was finally getting. The extra layer of body fat that was difficult to get rid of was finally coming off. I wasn't tired and exhausted after my run anymore. I was feeling less fatigue during the day and realized I had been over-training. After a few months of proper aerobic training, I began to notice I was running faster while at the same time keeping my heart rate below the 70% aerobic threshold. It was then that I started to appreciate the value of training at the proper intensity level (aerobic threshold). Not only did this new training regimen give me better physical fitness, it gave me better health. Remember, anaerobic training is stress producing and could be another straw on your camel's back, which can lead to further adrenal exhaustion.

The Heart Rate Monitor

We need to find out if we are training in our target fat-burning zone by first measuring our heart rates. The best and most accurate way to do this is with a heart rate monitor. They can be purchased at any local sporting goods store for less than a hundred dollars. The heart rate monitor consists of a transmitter and receiver. The transmitter is a band that you wear across your chest and is designed to pick up your heartbeat. It will then send a signal to the receiver. The receiver is designed as a wristwatch that is worn while you train. The purpose of the heart rate monitor is to measure your level of intensity as you train. It is a great investment and I wouldn't do my aerobic training without one.

The next step is to determine your target fat-burning zone or aerobic threshold. The old equation of subtracting your age from 220 and then multiplying that number by 55%, 70%, or 85% of your maximum heart rate does not take into consideration variables such as training history, weight, and health condition. You also need to have a calculator handy.

A simple and more accurate way to determine your aerobic threshold (target fat-burning zone) was designed by Dr. Phil Maffetone. It's called the 180-Formula, and he found that if you subtract your age from 180 (180 minus age equals Target Fat-Burning Zone), that number would be the high end of your target fat burning zone. This is approximately 70% of your maximum heart rate. For example, if someone were 40 years of age (180 minus 40 equals 140), he or she would not train above 140 bpm. This would be his or her aerobic threshold.

When we try to consider some of the variables we discussed earlier in regard to determining your aerobic threshold, Dr. Maffetone's 180-Formula takes into consideration some variables that need to be assessed. Two 40-year-old twins can't train at the same intensity level or heart rate and expect to get the same results if they have different training backgrounds. Oftentimes I see patients who walk or jog together, which is good, but they are at different levels of fitness. It's likely one person is in better condition than the other, and they should be walking at different speeds. One person may be exercising within his or her aerobic threshold while the other one isn't. This is why it is important to use a heart rate monitor when you train. You may not be aware that you are training too fast.

After you have subtracted your age from 180 you may need to add or subtract another 5 or 10 more points, depending on the history of this 40-year-old person.

• Subtract your age from 180 (180 minus age equals Aerobic Threshold).

• Modify this number by selecting one of the following categories:

If you have or are recovering from a major illness (heart disease, any operation, any hospital stay, etc.), or if you are on any regular medication

subtract 10.

If you have not exercised before, if you have been exercising but have been injured or are regressing in your training or competition, if you often get colds or flu, or if you have allergies

subtract 5.

If you have been exercising for up to two years without any real problems, and if you have not had colds or flu more than once or twice per year

subtract 0.

If you have been exercising for more than two years without any problems, while making progress in competition, without injury

add 5.

The classic complaint I receive from people who have just started using a heart rate monitor to keep track of their intensity levels are: "I can't work out this slow," and "Am I getting any benefits from going this slow?" The hardest thing is to get people to slow down. A rule of thumb to think about is: if you have to run at a very slow pace to stay below your aerobic threshold, I don't think you're in excellent aerobic condition. If your heart is racing at 80% of its maximum heart rate, but your little legs are only moving at 30% of your maximum speed, that's not good. The goal should be to have your heart beat at 70% of its maximum and have your muscles working at 70% of their maximum.

Patient Story

Joan was 54 when she began walking with her neighbors every morning. Her neighbors had been walking for some time and kept the pace fairly quick when they walked. After a couple of months walking every morning with her friends, she still hadn't lost any weight.

I felt her diet needed only a little adjustment, but for the most part it was working well for her. I suggested she get a heart rate monitor and not let her heart rate get above 125 bpm when she walked, and if it did she needed to slow down and walk at a pace that would keep her below her aerobic threshold. The next day when she walked with her neighbors, she noticed that her heart was racing at 140 bpm when she walked. Joan didn't like the idea of walking by herself or walking that slowly in order to keep her heart rate below 125 bpm, but she did, and within a couple of weeks she finally started to lose a few pounds. It seemed that Joan's friends were walking at a pace that was too fast for her.

A common mistake I often see is couples walking or jogging together, which is great for company and encouragement; however, one person is usually in better condition than the other, which means that person is getting a better aerobic workout and is building his or her aerobic capacity, while the other is not. This is why it's so important to be able to monitor your own intensity level, so you can train at the level that is beneficial for your body.

My Mother's Story

I want to share my mother's story because it is very typical of what most patients and athletes I have helped train experience. My mother, at age 60, had for the last few years been a steady walker and now had become a competitive race walker. She, in fact, had won so many trophies that she had taken down most of the trophies my brothers and I had won as kids to make room for hers. As well as she was doing, she was still carrying a little extra weight and I told her (very nicely) that the problem could be her training intensity.

I convinced her to start training with a heart rate monitor and found out she was training at a heart rate of 138 bpm. That is over 86% (220 minus 60 equals 160; 138 divided by 160 is 86%) of her maximum heart rate. Only well-conditioned marathoners and triathletes can exercise aerobically at 80–85% of their maximum heart rates and still be able to burn calories from stored body fat. Unfortunately, my mother was not a trained marathoner or triathlete, yet was trying to train as if she was. She was far above her aerobic threshold, which is one of the reasons she was unable to burn that extra weight off.

I told her she needed to walk at or below her aerobic threshold, which was determined using the 180-Formula. Her aerobic threshold was 120 bpm (180 minus 60 equals 120). She complained, said that it was too slow to walk at this speed, and felt she would not receive any health benefits.

With the aid of a treadmill, she started walking at or below 120 bpm. I let her know she could walk as fast as she wanted to as long as she kept her heart rate at or below 120 bpm. She initially started training at a speed of 2.5 miles per hour. After two weeks, she noticed that she had to increase her speed to 2.7 mph to keep her heart rate at or below 120 bpm. Within a couple more weeks, she now had to walk at a speed of 3.1 mph to keep her heart rate at or below 120 bpm. A few weeks later it was up to 3.4 mph; 3.8 mph; 4.1 mph. She finally started smiling! Eventually she started walking at 4.5 mph at 120 bpm. She expanded her aerobic capacity and found that to increase her heart rate up to 120 bpm she would have to increase her intensity and walk faster.

She was again walking at her original speed, but this time her heart was only beating 120 bpm instead of 138 bpm. Since her aerobic capacity increased, her body's ability to transport oxygen to her muscles became more efficient. Her heart didn't have to beat so fast to do the same amount of work as it did before. In reality, we decreased the stress she was placing on her heart because her heart muscles did not have to pump as much. Now when she trains, more of her aerobic metabolism is triggered than her anaerobic metabolism, which allows her body to finally burn calories from fats when she exercises.

The hardest part for my mother and most patients and athletes to understand is that we may have been training too hard or at too high of an intensity level. It is very difficult to convince someone, especially an athlete, to slow down with his or her intensity level when he or she trains. People are still believing and following the old battle cry of "No Pain, No Gain."

Aerobic Capacity

Training within your aerobic threshold increases your aerobic capacity, which is the maximum amount of work (exercise) the body can do and still provide oxygen to the muscles. As you consistently train below your aerobic threshold, you steadily expand your aerobic capacity.

The best way to explain how our aerobic capacity functions is to imagine your red blood cells as little trucks, with cargo beds for carrying oxygen. Does your truck have a large or small carrying capacity for oxygen? The larger the carrying capacity, the easier it is to transport and supply oxygen. The more you train aerobically, the larger your truck's carrying capacity becomes. If each truck can carry more oxygen because you are more aerobically fit, you don't need to send as many trucks. The trucks are dispatched by the heart with each heartbeat. Therefore, if the trucks have a small carrying capacity, more trucks need to be sent, as opposed to someone whose trucks have a larger carrying capacity because of proper aerobic training. This explains why a well-conditioned person has a lower heartbeat than an untrained or poorly conditioned person. His or her aerobic capacity has increased, making the heart need to work less. This is more efficient for the heart because it doesn't have to beat as much. Therefore, expanding our aerobic capacity contributes tremendously to our overall good health and fitness.

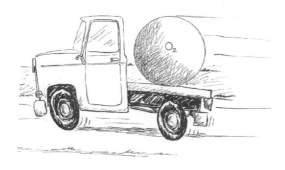

How big is your aerobic capacity?

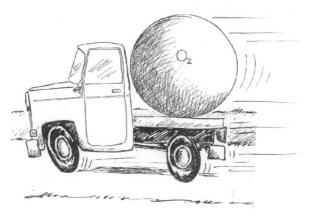

If you train at an intensity level that takes you above your aerobic threshold, you don't increase the oxygen-carrying capacity of those little trucks. Anaerobic training increases your body's ability to operate under anaerobic conditions, but since we spend approximately 23 hours a day in our aerobic systems, wouldn't it be smarter to train our aerobic systems and expand our aerobic capacity? The goal is to increase aerobic capacity. We do this by training aerobically 3–4 times a week. If we train aerobically anywhere from 20–60 minutes per workout, we expand our aerobic capacity.

Measuring Your Progress

Once you have determined your aerobic threshold, it will be important to measure your speed over time. If you determine your aerobic threshold is 140 bpm, you must do your aerobic training at an intensity level that keeps your heart rate at or below 140 bpm. To determine how much better your aerobic capacity becomes, you need to measure your training. The best way to do this is to go out to a local track or mark off a certain distance in your neighborhood. Measure how long it takes to walk or jog a few miles or how far around the block you can travel for 30 or 40 minutes at your aerobic threshold of 140 bpm.

Let's say it takes 30 minutes to walk or jog three miles at or below 140 bpm. Continue this exercise routine 3–4 times a week at this same intensity rate. One month later, go back and measure your time to walk or jog that same distance. The time it will take to cover this same distance at the same target heart rate may only take 29 minutes. This is because your aerobic capacity has increased; you increased the oxygen-carrying capacity. Continue doing the same routine for another month, while staying below the target fat-burning zone of 140 bpm. It may now take only 28 minutes to do the exact same distance that used to take 30 minutes. This is a typical example of the benefits someone will receive from training in his or her target fat-burning zone. The intensity level (heart rate) remains the same, yet your speed has increased. This progression will continue to occur as you train in this manner.

Summary

- Aerobic threshold is the maximum amount of intensity you can train at and have oxygen available.
- Well-conditioned athletes (marathoners and triathletes) can train at 80–85% of their maximum heart rates and still be aerobic.
- Most people need to train at around 70% of their maximum heart rates to stay aerobic.
- The 180-Formula subtracts your age from 180 to find your aerobic threshold.
- Increasing your aerobic capacity improves health and fitness.

Action Steps

- Determine your aerobic threshold with the 180-Formula.
- Monitor your heart rate with a heart rate monitor.
- Measure your aerobic capacity over time and distance and check it each month to see your progress.
- Begin training aerobically.

Chapter Nine

Exercising for Weight Loss and Fitness

The best type of exercise or workout you can choose to follow is a workout you like doing and will continue to do on a regular basis. It's best to get a combination of both aerobic and anaerobic (weight training) exercise in your day. There is not necessarily one exercise that is better than another. The best exercise to do is something you enjoy doing. If you hate to jog, your workout should not include jogging because you will probably not continue that regimen for very long. If you enjoy playing basketball, tennis, or soccer and would rather do that than jog, excellent. If you like to bike, rollerblade, or jump on a trampoline, these and any other type of physical activities that bring enjoyment and health benefits are excellent. Pick any physical activities you enjoy doing; chances are you will continue to incorporate those activities into your lifestyle. Don't buy a treadmill or stair-stepper to place in your house and use it only to hang clothes on.

The reason most of us are forced to follow some type of exercise program is because this is the only physical activity we get in our lives. For the last several thousand years, nobody really exercised except for athletes. We can attribute the decline of our daily physical activity to the Industrial Revolution, because everyone was getting enough exercise from his or her daily activities. Back then, we had no cars, we walked all the time, we carried things to and fro, and most of us worked the land. With those kinds of activities and demands, who needed to be spending additional time in a gym, working out?

Today, most people work out and exercise out of vanity, not because of the health benefits derived from exercise. The driving force behind our workout routines is to look and feel better! If that helps your heart, lowers blood pressure, keeps cholesterol down, keeps blood sugar under control, reduces arthritic pain, makes you look younger, keeps your belt or dress size from getting any larger, fantastic! Many of us are working out simply because of the weight we've gained, the muscles we've lost, or the muscles we've never had. We want to look and feel better about ourselves. Those are the real reasons people are exercising. If that sounds like you, let's make sure you get the most out of all the time, energy, and effort you spend working out.

Balancing Aerobic and Anaerobic Training

As I said before, good fitness and good health are two separate things. Let the facts be known: you can be in good shape physically, look great, and still be in poor overall health.

To achieve your weight loss goal and add muscle tone and shape to your body, it is important to do a combination of both aerobic and anaerobic training (strength training). *At least 50–70% of your training time should be dedicated to aerobic activities. The other 30–50% of your time should include anaerobic (strength and resistance) exercises.* This type of balance between aerobic and anaerobic activities will promote optimum health and fitness. Those who are poorly conditioned should strive to do more aerobic training (70%). If you're trying to add more shape to your body, I recommend a workout that is more evenly balanced between aerobic and anaerobic training.

More often than not, people do more of one type of training than the other. They may do more aerobic training and not enough anaerobic training, or just the opposite: too much anaerobic training compared to aerobic training. The key is to get a balance of both training activities into your busy schedule. Not to be gender specific, but oftentimes men prefer to lift weights and ignore the importance of including aerobic training, whereas women will often choose to do more aerobic training and leave out the strength training. Both types of training are valuable for overall good health and fitness.

In the earlier chapters, we discussed the importance of exercise to stimulate our metabolism. Exercise causes your metabolism to increase, which triggers the burning of additional calories. It doesn't matter if it is aerobic or anaerobic exercise; both will increase your metabolism. The reason for this is simple. Muscle tissue is metabolically more active than adipose tissue (fat). A pound of muscle burns more calories than a pound of fat! Therefore, you should be looking for ways to exercise the muscles of your body to help stimulate your metabolism. Are you using your muscles to keep your metabolism stimulated, or do you only use your muscles to walk from the bed to the bathroom, to the kitchen, to the car, to the elevator, back to the car, to the sofa, and back to bed? If that is the case, how are you expending any calories in the day, and how can you expect to raise your metabolism if you don't stimulate your muscles?

When you start to include exercise in your daily lifestyle, you are making your muscles work and are creating additional muscle tissue. Please don't think that weight training will immediately give you the look of the Incredible Hulk. That will take years of dedicated training and dieting. However, the additional muscle mass (muscle tissue) that is being stimulated will burn more calories for fuel than adipose tissue. So, if you can add more lean muscle tissue and/or require your muscles to do more activity throughout the day, the body burns more calories. Remember, you can achieve your goal of losing weight and keeping the weight off with a good diet. However, if your desire is to add some shape and tone to your body, you're going to have to do some strength training to complement your aerobic training.

Creating the Workout

The first thing you need to do is create a workout plan. Figure out how much time you can devote to exercising in a week. Can you work out three or five days a week? Do you have 30 minutes or an hour to work out in a day? Will you combine both aerobic and anaerobic training in a day? What aerobic activity do you plan on doing? What type of weight training routine will you follow? A good exercise program to promote better fitness (weight loss) and better health begins with aerobic training. At least 50–70% of your training time should be spent doing aerobic activities.

Secondly, figure out what your aerobic threshold or target fat-burning zone is. Use the 180-Formula. Many people are going to be surprised at how much slower they will have to perform their aerobic workouts, but as you consistently train within your aerobic threshold, your speed will gradually increase. Remember, it is only those well-conditioned athletes (marathoners and triathletes) who can train at up to 85% of their maximum heart rates and still depend on aerobic metabolism, so if you're not one of them it's probably better to keep your heart rate between 65–75% of your maximum heart rate.

Third, start exercising on a regular basis! Whether the exercise is walking, jogging, cycling, dancing, stair-climbing, swimming, skating, or boxing, it must be done on a continual basis. Working out one day a week is not going to give you the results you want. You need to make a commitment to yourself and be consistent with yourself.

Aerobic training should be done 3–5 times per week. If you are new to the idea of exercising and have never incorporated exercise into your lifestyle, begin training only three days per week for a minimum of 10–15 minutes each day. An eventual goal may be to exercise at least 3–5 days per week for a minimum of 30–60 minutes, aerobically.

Those of us who complain how boring and unpleasant aerobic training (jogging, cycling, swimming, or in-line skating) is may be pleasantly surprised, as I was when I finally started training properly. I know that when I used to train outside my target fat-burning zone, I would finish my workout happy that I was done but oftentimes not feeling great. I was typically exhausted from pushing myself too hard during the workout. Now when I finish my run, biking, or blading in my target fat-burning zone, I don't feel exhausted and tired. In fact, I feel quite refreshed when I am done. If you're not feeling refreshed when you finish your aerobic exercise, you are probably training at too high an intensity level and adding additional stress to an already exhausted body.

Progressive Resistance Training

Weight training or progressive resistance training is considered an anaerobic activity. Incorporating this type of training will help you reach the other part of your goal of shaping and toning your body.

Over the past 20-plus years of weight training, I have noticed that people who are trying to shape and tone the body oftentimes don't start with a good, fundamental routine that will get the most for the amount of time, energy, and effort spent lifting weights. If you are new to weight training or are not getting the results from your present weight training routine, let's get back to the basics.

To promote good fitness and good health, resistance training (strength training) should be 30–50% of our exercise time. Because time is so valuable for many of us, you must make sure that the exercises you choose will lead you to your goals as quickly as possible. Is your training time limited? Do you need to do four or five sets for each body part? Should you do exercises that work more than one muscle at a time?

Based solely on time, which is a major factor in determining if we can squeeze exercise into our busy lives, it would be advantageous to do exercises that incorporate multiple muscles for each exercise. What is meant by multiple muscle action is simple. If someone is doing bicep curls or triceps kickbacks to firm up the upper arms, he or she is doing an isolated movement that is specifically done to target one specific muscle. An example of an exercise that is considered a multiple muscle exercise is the push-up. The primary muscles involved in doing a pushup are the muscles of the chest, shoulders, and triceps. In fact, 60–70% of the stress from the pushup is targeted to the chest, 15–20% is targeted to the shoulders, and another 15–20% is targeted to the triceps. Understanding this makes it apparent why you should choose exercises that utilize multiple muscles, rather than exercises that isolate a single muscle, especially if time is a consideration.

A second rule of resistance training that should be observed is to train and exercise the larger muscles of the body first. The thigh muscles are larger than the calf muscles. The back muscles are larger than the bicep muscles. The chest muscles are bigger than the shoulder muscles, which are bigger than the triceps muscles, which are bigger than our bicep muscles.

It's wise to design a routine that takes the size of the muscles being exercised into consideration. The reason we want to make sure we exercise and train the larger muscles first is simple. The larger muscles fatigue and exhaust the body faster when you work them, compared to the smaller muscles. Therefore, don't try and do your leg workout at the end of your routine, because you may already be tired and those larger leg muscles will deplete what little energy you have left. Train the larger muscles first, when your energy level is at its highest. It doesn't take a lot of energy to do a set of bicep curls, but it does take a lot of energy to do a set of squats or pushups.

When you exercise the larger muscles, you burn more calories! This is why you want to make sure you spend more time working the larger muscles of your body, such as your legs, chest, and back. Since our larger muscles are made up of more muscle fibers and tissues, they require more energy in order to function. Energy is derived from burning calories. Therefore, the larger muscles will be metabolically more active (burn more calories) than smaller muscles throughout the day.

Stress and Weight Training

The effects of stress on our bodies are far-reaching. When you are constantly producing more cortisol in response to stress, you will be interfering with any muscle growth that you're after. Since cortisol promotes the breakdown of protein (lean muscle tissue), how do you expect your body to get the shape and tone you're after, if you are constantly triggering your stress hormones to break down muscles? The lack of results you are after with your weight training may be due to the excess production of cortisol, due to all the stress in your life. This is another reason why you must pay attention to your adrenal glands and the level of stress in your life.

If you feel that you are in Stage Two or Three of adrenal exhaustion, it would be wise to keep the stress to a minimum. You don't want to be placing any additional physical stress on your body. Therefore, it is wise to eliminate weight training for a short while, until your body is well rested and you are able to handle a taxing weight-training routine. If you are constantly exhausted, adding another physical stress to your camel's back is only going to make it worse. Limit your workouts only to aerobic training, which is stress reducing, until you properly rest, nourish your adrenal glands, and overcome your exhaustion. Hopefully, within 4–8 weeks you should be able to return to your weight-training workout, as long as you take the necessary steps and reduce the stress load in your life.

Summary

- 50–70% of exercise time should include aerobic training.
- 30–50% of exercise time should include anaerobic training.
- Muscle is metabolically more active than adipose (fat) tissue.
- Stimulating your muscles with exercise will increase your metabolism.
- Exercise the larger muscles first.
- Cortisol promotes the breakdown of lean muscle tissue.

Action Steps

- Determine how much time per week you can exercise.
- Divide your workouts into aerobic and anaerobic activities.
- Exercise at least three times per week.

Chapter Ten

The Super Seven Workout

Let me show you a very simple and effective workout routine that will give you the shape and tone you want for all the time, energy, and effort you spend working out. *The Super Seven Workout* combines aerobic and anaerobic exercises that will help you lose weight, add shape to your body, and most importantly improve your overall health. First, realize you don't have to train in a gym in order to do progressive resistance training. I will demonstrate exercises that can be done at home that will shape up the whole body. In fact, I typically train at home and only use my body weight for resistance. The workout I have outlined is pretty much all I do in order to stay in shape.

If you have a set of weights or access to a gym, you can do the same workout I've outlined. This workout is meant to work all the major muscles of the body. It is also chosen because it incorporates many muscles per each movement and can be done in as little as 15 minutes, three times a week.

Leg Squats—target the large muscles of the thigh and buttock.
Toe Touches—exercise the hamstring and lower back.
Calf Raises—work the calf muscles.
Push-Ups or Bench Presses—a pushing motion that targets the chest muscles as well as the shoulders and triceps.
Pull-Ups or Cable Rows—a pulling movement that exercises the back, biceps, and forearm muscles.
Abdominal Crunches—target the abdominal muscles.

There are many other exercises that can be incorporated into your routine. These six fundamental exercises completely work all the major muscles of your body in the shortest amount of time. Let's explain why these six exercises completely train every major muscle group of the body.

Leg Squats—work the largest group of muscles on the body. We want to work them first. Leg squats work all the muscles of the thigh and buttock. A leg press and leg extension machine can be used instead of doing squats. The leg extension machine only targets the thigh muscles and does not stimulate the buttocks. Whether you train at home or in a gym you can do leg squats, with or without additional weight. Lunges can be substituted or alternated for leg squats. I typically do leg squats without weight and do 50–80 repetitions per set.

Toe Touches—will target the hamstring (muscles on the back of the thigh) and lower back. They can be done with or without additional weight. Those who have access to a leg curl machine can replace toe touches with leg curls.

Calf Raises—work the powerful muscles of the lower leg. If you train at home and want to increase the intensity, you can either hold a hand weight or do calf raises one leg at a time. I recommend doing calf raises on a step, which allows for greater range of motion.

Push-Ups or Bench Presses—develop half of the major muscles of the upper body. This "pushing" movement is a foundational exercise because it works half the muscles of the upper body. The muscles of the chest, shoulders, and triceps are exercised when any type of pushing motion is performed. If you prefer to work out at home, do push-ups. If you work out in a gym, you can do bench press with either a barbell or a dumbbell. Machines that simulate the same pushing movement can be utilized. Modified (kneeling) push-ups are a great way to lower the resistance for those of us who are unable to perform 8–12 repetitions.

Pull-Ups or Cable Rows—this "pulling" motion develops the other half of the major muscles of the upper body. When you do a pull-up or rowing movement you exercise the muscles of the back, biceps, and forearms. Doing a pull-up may be quite difficult for many of us. Therefore, you can do what I call "modified pull-ups." In your doorway or at your gym, place a bar about three feet off the ground and pull yourself up, while your feet remain flat on the ground. The purpose of the modified pull-up is that it allows those who are unable to pull their own body weight up for 8–12 repetitions to off-load 25–35% of their body weight, and successfully perform 8–12 repetitions. It is a lot like doing a modified push-up. Rubber tubing can be used to perform this movement at home. If you exercise in a gym, I recommend doing either seated cable rows or seated pull-downs. Both work the muscles of the back, biceps, and forearms.

Abdominal Crunches—strengthen your midsection. They can be done anywhere and will help support the lower back. This movement isolates the muscles of the abdomen by specifically targeting only those muscles.

Secondary Exercises

Shoulder Presses—target the shoulder and triceps muscles.
Upright Rows—target the shoulder and bicep muscles.
Triceps Press-Downs—isolate the triceps muscles.
Bicep Curls—isolate the bicep muscles.
Wrist Curls and Reverse Wrist Curls—exercise the muscles of the forearm.

Shoulder Presses—are a powerful pushing motion that strengthens and develops the shoulders and triceps. This overhead pushing motion can be performed with a barbell, dumbbell, machine, or elastic bands.

Upright Rows—are a pulling exercise that targets the shoulder muscles along with the bicep muscles. This pulling motion can be done with a dumbbell, barbell, cable, or elastic bands.

Triceps Press-Downs—isolate the triceps muscles.

Bicep Curls—target the bicep muscles.

Wrist Curls and Reverse Wrist Curls—target the forearm muscles.

The secondary exercises should only be done after the basic movements have been completed.

How Much and How Often?

The best methods of increasing muscle strength and tone are with progressive resistance (weight training). The reason it is called progressive resistance is that we must progressively increase the intensity level of our workouts in order to stimulate the muscles to become stronger and firmer.

The intensity level can be increased in one of three ways. First, add more weight to the exercise. The second way is to add more repetitions to the exercise, and the last is to decrease the amount of rest between each set. Whichever is chosen, the intensity level will be increased, which places more stress on the muscles and causes them to become stronger and firmer.

Performing these basic exercises 2–3 times per week is all you need to do to get the shape you're after. Now you need to figure out how many repetitions, how many sets, and how much weight you should be lifting. A simple rule of thumb to follow when using weights is to perform 8–12 repetitions per set for upper body muscles, and 15–20 repetitions for lower body muscles. If you are using your body weight as resistance, the number of repetitions can be much higher.

A repetition is the number of times you complete a particular movement from start to finish. For example, if you do 10 push-ups, you are doing one set of 10 repetitions. If you wait a minute after doing the first 10 push-ups and do another 10 push-ups, wait another minute and do another 10 push-ups, you would have completed three sets of 10 repetitions of push-ups.

A second suggestion would be to do 3–4 sets of a particular exercise for the larger muscles (legs, chest, and back) and 1–2 sets for the smaller muscles (shoulders, triceps, and biceps). Always remember: our larger muscles can do more work than our smaller muscles, and the smaller muscles are usually involved in exercises for the larger muscles. These smaller muscles, such as triceps and biceps, are getting exercised when they assist in the pushing or pulling movement. Therefore, you don't need to overwork these smaller muscles with the same number of sets that you would for the larger muscles.

The amount of weight you should use is fairly simple to figure out. Use the amount of weight you can lift for no more than 8–12 repetitions. If you are doing bench press, you should be lifting as much weight as you can, so that you are unable to perform more than 8–12 repetitions. When you are able to successfully perform 8–12 repetitions on the bench press, it is now time to add more weight, do more repetitions, or decrease your rest period to continually stress the muscles.

Progressive resistance is needed in order to stimulate your muscles to become firmer and stronger. You do not stress the muscles to become any firmer or stronger if you do 8–12 repetitions and stop, when you could have done 15–20 repetitions. This is an important sticking point for many of us who exercise and aren't seeing results.

What Is Your Weight Training Intensity?

One of the biggest mistakes I see people making in a gym is using the wrong weight when they exercise. For muscles to become firmer and stronger, we need to challenge and stress them. We need to continually make the muscles work harder to stimulate them; otherwise they won't change and they'll stay the same. What I typically see is someone doing an exercise, let's say bench press, and they are doing 10 repetitions and stopping. It is acceptable to do 10 repetitions if the tenth repetition was the last one that you could possibly perform. However, most people will stop after 10 repetitions when they could have actually done 15–20 repetitions. When they do that, they never stress the muscles or stimulate them to become stronger and firmer.

How will your muscles shape up, if they are not being challenged? If the muscles can already lift the weight 10 times, they don't need to become any stronger or firmer than they already are. If you want to add more tone to your body, you need to stimulate the muscles in order to make them change.

Think of it this way. If you stop at 10 repetitions when you can actually do 20 repetitions with the same weight, you never recruit additional muscle fibers to come into action. It is as if the muscles of your body are saying, "I don't need to get any firmer or stronger because I can already handle that amount of weight that you want me to lift." However, if you make your muscles work harder by lifting heavier weights, doing more repetitions, or decreasing your rest period, you now begin to challenge and stress those muscles. The muscles respond and adapt to that stress and become stronger and firmer.

Don't get the wrong idea that you will soon begin looking like Mr. or Ms. Universe if you stress your muscles this way. I am suggesting you train at an intensity level to get the results you seek for the time, energy, and effort spent. If you don't stress your muscles to do more than they can already do, there is no reason for them to adapt and become any stronger or firmer.

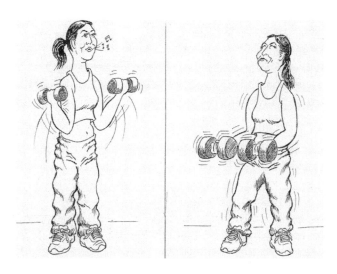

Does your training intensity stimulate muscle growth?

Patient Story

Susan was 43 years old and enjoyed working out six days a week. She would walk three times a week and lift weights three times a week. Her main complaint was that she never as if she was firming her body when she lifted weights. When I reviewed her training intensity, I found out that when she lifted weights, she never lifted enough weight to stress or stimulate her muscles. Part of her workout included ten-pound dumbbell curls, 20-pound bench presses and 40-pound leg presses.

I asked her how many repetitions she was doing and how difficult it was to complete a set. She said she would do 15–20 repetitions on all her exercises and the weights never felt heavy. She told me she could do more weight, but was afraid that she would get bulky. I explained how muscles respond to stress and how they need to be stressed in order for them to become firmer and stronger.

On her next visit to the gym, she took my advice and increased her intensity. She now performed 10–15 repetitions for the smaller upper body muscles and 15–20 repeitions for the larger lower body muscles. The next day she called and said it was the first time she actually felt sore after a weight-training workout. She kept up with her intensity level, and six weeks later was able to notice a difference with her muscle tone.

I am not saying that you need to be "busting a gut" or hurting yourself on every repetition. What I am saying is that it is important to stimulate the muscles. This happens by making certain the last couple of repetitions are difficult to perform. Otherwise, you may not be stimulating any type of muscle growth to occur and are basically spinning your wheels. Examine your intensity level; do you use the proper weights in order to stimulate muscle growth? Are you progressively increasing the resistance in your workout? If you're not, you need to increase the intensity level of your workout.

The Super Seven Workout

This is a simple and effective workout designed to stimulate weight loss, increase muscle tone, and improve your overall health. The principles behind the workout make it the most efficient and effective training routine for the amount of time, energy, and effort spent exercising. If you can devote only three days a week for 45 minutes to an hour to work out, here is a simple routine that will give you the results we have been talking about.

The first part of *The Super Seven Workout* is 30 minutes of any type of aerobic training (pick your exercise: walk, jog, cycle, stairs-climb, in-line skate, swim, etc.). This aerobic activity must be done below your aerobic threshold, which is determined by the 180-Formula.

The second part of *The Super Seven* is the six strength-training exercises. These primary or core exercises will work all the major muscles of the body and can be done in as little as 15 minutes, three times a week.

3–4 sets of leg squats
2–3 sets of toe touches
2–3 sets of calf raises
3–4 sets of push-ups or bench presses
3–4 sets of pull-ups or cable rows
1–2 sets of as many crunches as you can do

The number of repetitions for each exercise will be different, depending on whether or not you work out at home or have access to a gym. Whatever the case, remember to do 8–12 repetitions for the upper body and 15–20 repetitions for the lower body, if you train with weights. Progressively increase the resistance by either adding more weight, increasing the number of repetitions, or decreasing the amount of rest between sets.

The Super Seven Workout

	Without weights	*With weights*
Leg Squats	25–75 reps	15–20 reps
Toe Touches	20–30 reps	15–20 reps
Calf Raises	20–50 reps	15–20 reps
Push-Ups	10–30 reps	-------
Bench Presses	-------	8–12 reps
Hanging Pull-Ups	10–30 reps	-------
Cable Rows	-------	8–12 reps

50–100 Abdominal Crunches

With time permitting in your workout schedule, you are at liberty to add to *The Super Seven* and target the specific smaller muscles with some of the secondary exercises mentioned below.

1 set of shoulder presses
1 set of shoulder shrugs
1 set of triceps press-downs
1 set of bicep curls
1 set of reverse wrist curls
1 set of wrist curls

Each of these exercises should be done with 8–12 repetitions.

The most important part of *The Super Seven Workout* is that you spend 50–70% of your time doing aerobic training. Secondly, you cannot add any of the secondary exercises until all of the six primary exercises are performed first. If time permits in your schedule, you can add the secondary exercises to your routine. Third, you don't need to perform more than 3–4 sets for the larger muscles, and only 1–2 sets for the smaller muscles.

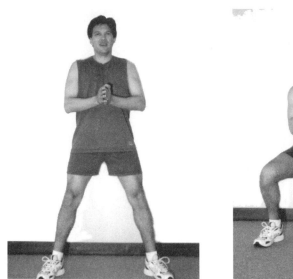
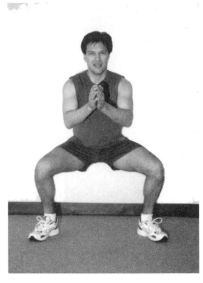

Squats—Begin with your feet flat on the floor, toes slightly pointed out. Bend the knees and lower yourself until the tops of your thighs are parallel to the floor. Keep your back straight.

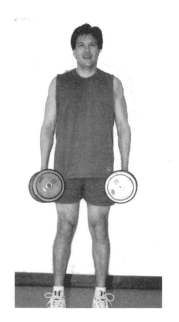
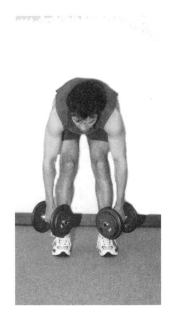

Toe Touches—Begin with your knees slightly bent, keep your back straight, and bend at the waist and lower yourself. Try to touch your toes or the tops of your ankles.

134

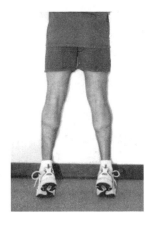

Calf Raises—With your toes slightly pointed out, rise up onto the balls of your toes, then lower yourself. If you can place the balls of your feet on a step, it will increase the stretch.

Push Movement

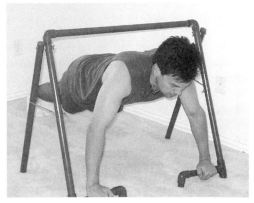

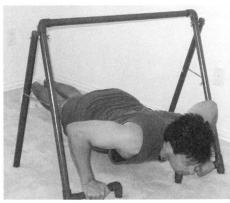

Push-Ups—Arms shoulder-width apart, lower yourself until you almost touch the ground with your chest. Modified push-ups with your knees on the ground will reduce the weight.

Pull Movement

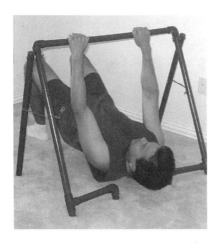 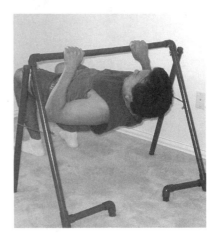

Hanging Pull-Ups—Start with the feet flat on the floor; arms are shoulder-width apart with an overhand grip. Hang yourself from a bar that is 30–36 inches off the ground. Pull yourself up until front of your chest almost touches the bar, then lower yourself.

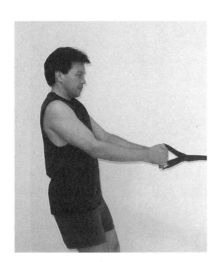 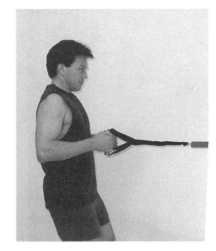

Wall Pulls—With knees slightly bent and arms extended, pull toward the chest and pull the shoulders back.

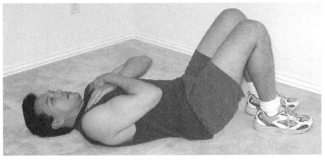

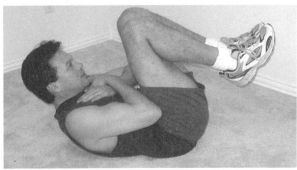

Abdominal Crunches—Start with your feet flat on the ground. Lay your arms across the chest or behind the head. At the same time, pull your knees to your chest and pull down toward your pelvis.

Secondary Exercises

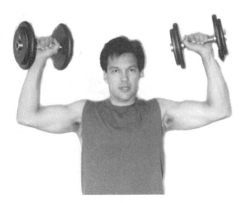

Overhead Presses—Press the weight overhead and then lower it to about eye level. This can be done either sitting or standing. Placing your elbows out to the side or the front will target the shoulder muscles differently.

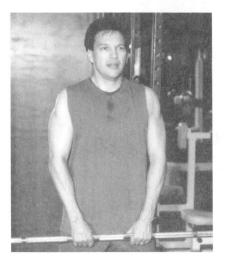
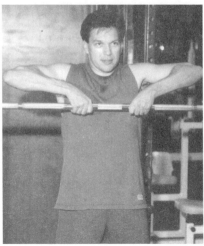

Upright Rows—Begin with your feet shoulder-width apart. With an overhand grip pull the barbell (dumbbell, cable, or elastic bands) up to your chin and then lower the bar. Keep your abdominals tight and limit the swing of the upper torso.

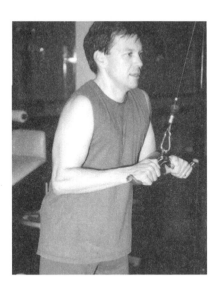
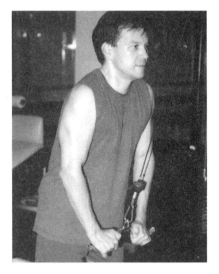

Tricep Push-Downs—Begin with your feet flat on the floor, shoulder-width apart. Grab the cable or elastic band with an overhand grip and push down, to straighten the arms. Control the weight when it comes back to the starting position until the arms are bent around 90 degrees, and then push on it.

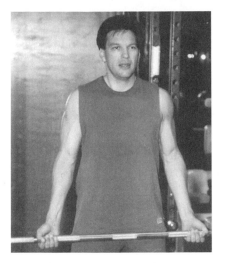 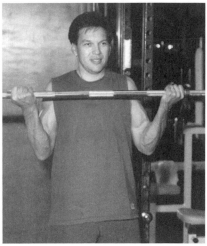

Bicep Curls—With feet flat on the ground, grab the bar with an underhand grip about shoulder-width apart. Tighten your back muscles and curl the bar (dumbbell, cable, or elastic bands). Do not rock or swing the body in order to do another repetition.

The Five- or-Six-Day Workout

For those who have more time available or are more eager to work out and are hoping to speed up their results, you can train five or six days. Here's how.

Monday, Wednesday, and Friday, train aerobically for 30 minutes to an hour. Tuesday, Thursday, and Saturday, weight train for 30 minutes to an hour.

Many times I find myself with only 30–45 minutes to train. When this is the case, I will do *The Super Seven Workout* in that time. I simply reduce the amount of time I train aerobically and reduce the number of sets from three to two. I attempt to keep the same proportions of 50–70% of my training as aerobic training and 30–50% of my time doing progressive resistance exercises.

Why the Super Seven Workout?

There are two reasons why I feel these seven exercises are all you need to do to achieve a physique that is leaner and firmer than you have now. First, all our military personnel in boot camp only do exercises that require their own body weight. They are not working out with weights, and they get in excellent physical condition by running and doing push-ups, pull-ups, and crunches.

Secondly, Herschel Walker, arguably one of the greatest collegiate running backs, who also had a very impressive and successful career with the Dallas Cowboys, was never known to lift weights. Many people may have heard the story that as a teenager, he would do hundreds of push-ups and sit-ups each day. He was known to have followed the same kind of routine as a collegiate as well as a professional athlete. Herschel Walker did not spend much time in the gym lifting weights, but by following his routine regularly he developed a physique that most people would envy.

With those two facts in mind, it should easily be recognized that you don't need to be in a gym in order to lose weight and shape up your body. You just have to make sure that you regularly work out, include both aerobic and anaerobic training, and diet accordingly to trigger your hormones to burn fat.

Training Tips

Start with a good pair of walking, running, or cross-training shoes. If you have a flat foot or high arch, it is important to wear proper shoes. If you have flat feet (pronator) or high arches (supinator), you should be wearing a shoe that is constructed to support the biomechanical movement for your specific feet. These two shoe designs are different. I see patients who complain of knee or hip pain that is caused by wearing the wrong shoes for their feet. Whenever you buy walking, running, or cross-training shoes, inform the sales clerk that you either have flat feet (pronator) or high arches (supinator).

If they don't know what you are talking about, find a more knowledgeable clerk or go to another store. Remember, the feet are the foundation of your body. A good shoe does not have to be an expensive shoe, but it does have to fit properly and move in accordance to how your foot moves.

Drink plenty of water before, during, and after your workout. It is recommended that we drink 8–10 glasses of water a day. If we add exercise to our daily lifestyle, we need to be drinking another couple of glasses. If you are constantly feeling thirsty, that is not a good sign. That is an indication that your body is in a state of dehydration. The body prefers water. Coffee, sodas, juices, and flavored drinks are not water. The kidneys have to work harder to separate the water from the rest of the contents. Also, all caffeinated drinks, such as coffee and most soft drinks, act as diuretics that cause us to urinate more often and lead to dehydration.

Warm up and lightly stretch before and after your workout. A good warm-up may consist of walking or riding a stationary bike for 5–10 minutes to get the blood flowing. One of the worst mistakes people make is stretching their cold muscles before they are warmed. Many times people arrive at the gym right after work, where they have been sedentary all day long. They usually proceed to the squat rack or bench press and quickly tug on their legs or shoulders to stretch and warm up. Since the muscles are not warmed up and are cold and inelastic, they begin to microscopically tear those muscles as they tug and pull on their legs and arms. Think of your muscles as being like a rubber band. Have you ever tried to stretch a rubber band that has been left out in the cold? It doesn't stretch very well. In fact, it may snap and tear. This is what happens to our muscles. I think dancers have it figured out! They spend 10–15 minutes doing basic movements to warm up their muscles and then proceed to stretch.

Get plenty of sleep (7–9 hours) each night. This is when the body repairs and rebuilds. We recharge our "batteries" when we sleep. One of the simplest and most overlooked aspects of any exercise program is our sleep and recovery. If you are not getting adequate sleep each night, it will catch up with you and this could be why you may always be exhausted. If we don't let our bodies rest and repair, how in the world can we expect our bodies to grow and become stronger and firmer? When we sleep, our bodies release most of our growth hormones. If you don't allow your bodies to properly recover you may be compromising your immune system as well as limiting any type of benefits from your workouts. Up to 20% of the benefits from exercise come from rest and recuperation.

Don't work out after eating! If you do, you may be turning off the Resting/Digesting mode and turning on the Fight or Flight mode while there is still food in your tummy. If you are going to do some light aerobic exercise this should not be a problem. However, for intense weight-training workouts, sprints, spin, aerobic, or boxing classes, no food should be eaten for at least an hour before the workout. If you work out within an hour of eating a meal, your body may still be digesting the food. As soon as you start an intense workout, all the blood needed to digest your food will be rerouted to your muscles. This inhibits proper digestion and creates digestive problems such as bloating, gas, indigestion, and poor absorption of your nutrients.

Certain foods digest faster than others. Most fruits when eaten alone can digest in approximately 20–45 minutes. Starchy carbohydrates take longer to digest than fruits. Proteins and fats may take up to two hours or more to digest. Depending on what you ate before your workout, that will determine how long you should wait before doing any anaerobic training. Don't make the classic mistake and drink a protein drink before going to the gym, thinking that it will help you get through your workout. If you think you need a boost of energy to get through your workout after a long day, try some fruit. The fruit will digest rapidly and its sugar will be assimilated very quickly into energy, which is what you need to complete a good anaerobic workout. Some people who drink a protein drink prior to their workouts oftentimes complain of intestinal gas and bloating. The simple reason for this is that the protein has not been digested and is rotting and putrefying inside their stomachs. Another reason for all the intestinal gas and bloating could be the lack of digestive enzymes and hydrochloric acid, which is needed to properly break down and assimilate the protein in your meal. Still another reason can be poor food combinations. If you have a history of digestive difficulties, proper food combination is essential.

In Summary

To Burn or Not to Burn, Fat Is the Question!

In conclusion, as I stated on the cover of this book, are you burning or storing body fat? My goal at the beginning of this book was to look at some of the pieces of the puzzle that are being overlooked and could be responsible for all the weight gain and difficulty losing weight in our society.

I hope you now have a better understanding of how stress can affect your hormones and that excessive, chronic stress can create hormonal imbalances. These imbalances can be why you have not had the success you have been looking for in your weight loss efforts. Therefore, the stress you place on your body is one piece of the puzzle that needs to be looked at if you are not reaching your goals of losing weight and keeping it off.

Have you exhausted your adrenal glands so much that they are not letting your body burn calories from stored body fat?

A second piece of the puzzle you need to consider is your diet and blood sugar levels. Our food selections are therefore another piece of the puzzle that needs to be considered. When you begin to analyze your diet with the knowledge that some foods will trigger your body to store fats, while other foods trigger your body to burn fats, you need to make better decisions with your food selections and regulate your blood sugar more evenly to promote healthy weight loss.

The last piece of the puzzle is the intensity level of your exercise routine. If your intensity level is higher than it should be, this can affect the results you hope to gain from your training activities. If you want to shed some of the fat from your body and replace it with some lean muscle tissue, you must do the appropriate exercises at the proper intensity level to achieve these results. Look at the results you have achieved from your training program. The training intensity you work out at may be another piece of the puzzle that needs to be examined to achieve the results you want.

The puzzle as a whole, as I see it is how can you become healthier? As I first stated, good fitness starts with good health. When you examine all the pieces of the puzzle and work at bringing them back in balance, your health will improve. As your health improves, your body will not need to carry this extra weight, which is counterproductive and unhealthy. Therefore, I believe the success of any long-term weight loss program is based on triggering the body to continually burn calories from stored body fats. It's not just diet and exercise! Stress is an important player in the success or failure of your weight loss efforts.

You have learned that hormones regulate your body and that some hormones store fat and some can burn fat. You've learned that the level of stress in your life, the type of diet you follow, and the intensity of your workout can influence your hormones to work with you or against you. The key is to remember you ultimately have the control and can regulate which hormones will be more abundant in your body.

Finally, to those of you out there reading this information and who are about to start following some of the principles, it is important to realize that these are lifestyle commitments and changes that can have a very positive effect on your life. Realize that some days you may not diet the way we talked about, but tomorrow is another day. Each week, attempt to do more things that are positive for your health, rather than negative and destructive to your health. Are you taking more Action Steps forward than you are taking backward each week? If you are, fantastic! The goal is to always take more Action Steps forward in the right direction.

In Good Health,

Dr. Len Lopez

The End

Frequently Asked Questions

Q. If stress is the reason I am unable to lose weight, where do I begin?

A. If after adjusting your diet and exercise routine you are still unable to lose weight, review the seven different types of stress that tax your body and determine which ones need to be adjusted. If there is a large amount of emotional stress in your life, you need to find ways (counseling, meditation, prayer, deep breathing, biofeedback) to control and lower the effects stress has on your body. If there is a large amount of any of the other stresses (internal, microbial, chemical, physical, electromagnetic, or nutritional deficiencies), work to lower those stresses first, which will give you better health. When you are in better health it is easier to get rid of unnecessary weight.

Q. Is there a way to measure how stress affects my adrenal glands and my inability to burn fat and lose weight?

A. A 24-hour saliva test that measures both your cortisol and DHEA is an accurate way to measure the functional status of your adrenal glands. Four saliva samples are taken throughout the day and tested. I prefer this test instead of a blood test for two simple reasons. First, cortisol fluctuates throughout the day; therefore, one blood draw may not give as accurate a picture as four samples in a day. Secondly, the test can be done in the convenience of your own home. This eliminates the emotional stress and anxiety and worry of going to the doctor's office, which sometimes can alter the levels of your hormones.

Q. Why are cortisol and DHEA so important in a weight loss program?

A. Cortisol and DHEA levels are not only important for weight loss but are equally important in maintaining good health. When your body is under constant stress it produces cortisol. The constant production of cortisol triggers the body to burn calories from carbohydrates and proteins and inhibits the breakdown of stored body fats. The hormone

DHEA has a positive effect on your overall health. It has been found to help with building muscle, burning fat, regulating blood sugar, and increasing energy, vitality, libido, and mental sharpness.

Q. What is functional adrenal exhaustion?

A. It is a term to describe what the body goes through when it has been excessively taxed with constant stress for an extended amount of time. When you are always under constant stress, your body is constantly triggered to produce cortisol in order to protect itself. Your adrenal glands can only produce so much cortisol before they become depleted and exhausted. When this happens, the ability to lose weight becomes more difficult, and other health complaints can develop due to a weakened immune system, such as fatigue, food cravings, allergies, irritability, depression, inability to concentrate, insomnia, etc.

Q. If my adrenal glands are exhausted, what do I do to support them?

A. Once you've determined which type of stress is burdening your body and have begun to lower that stress, it is important to rest and nourish your adrenal glands. First, get plenty of sleep each day and supplement your diet with nutrients that support the adrenal glands, such as vitamin C, B-complex, pantothenic acid, zinc, magnesium, ginseng, licorice root, withania, cordyceps, and adrenal glandulars.

Q. I seem to constantly be bothered by indigestion, bloating, gas, heartburn, and constipation. Will this have an effect on my weight loss efforts?

A. Yes! If you are constantly bothered by these problems you are having a difficult time absorbing your nutrients and eliminating the poisons from your body. This can affect how well your body responds to a weight loss program. Digestive enzymes, good gut bacteria (probiotics), proper food combining, and a good natural fiber supplement can help with these symptoms. Once these symptoms are eliminated, your success on a weight loss program should increase.

Q. I've heard that a detoxification program can be helpful prior to starting a weight loss program. What is the purpose of a detoxification program?

A. A detoxification (detox) or cleansing program can be very helpful in a weight loss program. The purpose of a detox is to remove any harmful toxins that are in your body. I spoke of chemical stresses and how various toxins can interfere with the function of your body and your overall good health. Most detox programs last 2–4 weeks and are meant to flush out many of the toxins and poisons found in your liver, large intestines, lymphatics, and skin. The liver and large intestines are the major cleansing organs of the body. A diet loaded with processed food, junk food, pesticides, insecticides, antibiotics, preservatives, artificial sweeteners, prescription drugs, and toxins in water and the air we breathe all has an effect on the functional capabilities of these organs. A diet loaded with fresh fruits and vegetables helps to keep these organs clean, which improves your overall good health.

Q. Isn't it important to count calories and fat grams in a weight loss program?

A. For thousands of years we have lived without counting calories or fat grams and have never had the problem with obesity we do today. Of course, if you eat more calories than you burn each day, you run the risk of gaining weight. The goal is to eat a better ratio of carbohydrates to fats to proteins, in order to trigger your hormones to burn calories from stored body fat and not from lean muscle tissue.

Q. Is this just another low-carbohydrate diet?

A. No! The main emphasis in our dieting approach is to reduce the intake of refined carbohydrates in order to balance our blood sugar levels. For years consumers have been told that fats are the problem, and that we should eat no-fat or low-fat foods. Thus, the American diet has changed to include so much refined carbohydrates. Since a greater percentage of calories come from carbohydrates, we are triggering hormones to store calories rather than burn calories.

Q. How do carbohydrates, proteins, and fats affect my weight loss efforts?

A. A diet high in carbohydrates triggers the release of a hormone called insulin. A diet with fewer carbohydrates and more proteins and fats triggers the release of the hormone glucagon. Insulin inhibits the production of glucagon. Insulin triggers the body to store carbohydrates and fats, while glucagon triggers the body to burn fat. Therefore, it is important to have a meal that does not trigger a large release of the hormone insulin. Unfortunately, most of the calories in today's diet come from refined and processed carbohydrates, which cause a huge release of insulin.

Q. Do I need to exercise in order to lose weight and add some tone to my body?

A. Exercise will only complement your dieting efforts and speed up your results. If you are wanting to add some tone and shape to your body, you will need to include some exercise in your daily activities.

Q. How much time do I need to spend working out in order to lose weight?

A. Ideally, it would be great to exercise 3–5 times a week for 45 minutes to an hour. If you are only able to exercise three times a week for 30 minutes, that's a step in the right direction. The goal should be to start getting some physical activity in your life, in order to help stimulate your metabolism.

Q. I thought you had to exercise at least 20 minutes before your body is able to burn fat?

A. That's not true! Your body is always burning calories from a combination of fats, proteins, and carbohydrates. As you increase your exercise intensity (increased heart rate), you begin to burn more calories from carbohydrates and fewer from fats. It is when your exercise intensity level exceeds your "aerobic threshold" that you only burn calories from carbohydrates.

Q. What is the difference between aerobic and anaerobic exercise?

A. Aerobic exercises, such as walking, jogging, cycling, swimming, aerobic dance, in-line skating, etc., are
• Stress reducing to the body.
• Low to moderate intensity.
• Performed for long periods of time.
• With oxygen.

Anaerobic exercises such as weightlifting, sprinting, speed skating, etc., are
• Stress producing to the body.
• Higher intensity.
• Performed for short periods of time.
• Without oxygen.

Q. What is the difference between aerobic and anaerobic metabolism?

A. The difference is oxygen! "Aerobic" means with oxygen. "Anaerobic" means without oxygen. The human body has a couple of ways of producing energy. If there is oxygen (aerobic) present, the body is able to burn calories from fat. If there is no oxygen (anaerobic) available, the body is unable to burn calories from fat and is forced to burn calories from carbohydrates and proteins.

Q. How do I measure the intensity level for my aerobic workouts, and what will it tell me?

A. Your heart rate determines the intensity level of your workout. As you increase the speed of your walking, jogging, cycling, swimming, etc., your heart rate increases. As your intensity level increases, your availability of oxygen decreases. Oxygen is needed in order to burn calories from fat. If there is no oxygen available, the body is forced to use "anaerobic metabolism" and can only burn calories from carbohydrates and proteins. The intensity level you train at will let you know if you are burning calories from fats or carbohydrates. A heart rate monitor is a valuable tool that helps you monitor the intensity level of your aerobic training.

Q. Shouldn't I just concentrate on burning calories?

A. It is important to burn calories, but it is more important in a weight loss program to burn calories from stored body fat rather than from the foods you just ate earlier in the day. Wouldn't it be smarter to trigger your body to burn 300 calories from the breakdown of fats, as opposed to breaking down 300 calories from carbohydrates?

Q. What is the "aerobic threshold" and why should I want to train below it?

A. The aerobic threshold is the maximum amount of intensity you can train at and still have oxygen available in your body. It is also called your "fat-burning zone." When you train above your aerobic threshold (fat-burning zone), your body will only burn calories from carbohydrates and proteins. Therefore, in order to burn more calories from fats, it is important to train at an intensity level below your aerobic threshold. This allows oxygen to remain in your tissues, which triggers aerobic metabolism and the breakdown of fats for energy.

Q. How do I find my aerobic threshold?

A. The best formula to determine your aerobic threshold is called the 180-Formula. Subtract your age from 180, and let that be the maximum you let your heart beat when you train aerobically. Depending on your current health condition, you may need to adjust this number up or down 5 or 10 points. Most people need to train at or below 70% of their maximum heart rates. More details are found inside the book.

Q. How long should it take me to do a weight-training workout?

A. A good weight-training workout for people who are not competitive athletes should take less than one hour. A good intense workout with weights can be done in as little as 30 minutes, not including the time it takes to warm up and cool down. *The Super Seven Workout* is designed so you can do your strength-training routine in as little as 15 minutes a day, three times a week.

About the Author

Len Lopez, D.C., C.C.N.

Dr. Lopez began his career in Dallas, Texas as a doctor of chiropractic. With a desire to treat patients with natural, complementary medicine, he expanded his professional training and became a Certified Clinical Nutritionist (C.C.N.), Certified Chiropractic Sports Physician (C.C.S.P.), and Certified Strength and Conditioning Specialist (C.S.C.S.), with additional training in Applied Kinesiology (A.K.) and homeopathy. He is an Adjunct professor at Parker College of Chiropractic and was the host of the TV show *Natural Health Made Simple*. His approach to healing is very simple: "Treat the Cause—Not the Symptom." Dr. Lopez is an avid fitness enthusiast who shares his life with his wife, Melissa, and their two dogs, Sammy and Rudy.

References

Baechle, T. 1994. *Essentials of Strength Training & Conditioning.* Human Kinetics.

Guyton, A. 1991. *Textbook of Medical Physiology,* 8th ed. Saunders.

McArdle, Katch, FI & VL. 1996. *Exercise Physiology,* 4th ed. Williams & Wilkins.

Maffetone, P. 1999. *Complementary Sports Medicine.* Human Kinetics.

Murray, M., & Pizzorno, J. 1998. *Encyclopedia of Natural Medicine.* Prima.